Her Story To Tell

Deborah Manning

Copyright © 2012 Deborah Manning

All rights reserved.

ISBN: 9798883227096

DEDICATION

To my little Jojo,

*You are here to tell your own story,
and I am just the one to share it with the world,
for everyone should know about the incredible little girl
that I am lucky enough to call my daughter.*

*Forever proud of your strength and beauty
and eternally grateful you chose me to be your Mummy.*

Thank you for being perfectly you.

Mummy loves you, always.
xxx

ACKNOWLEDGMENTS

Shellie Wall Photography

Sarah Carter Photography

PROLOGUE

Most stories start at the beginning, but mine I am going to start at the end, the end that is really only the beginning. Because, if you only read one page of this book then I want you to know that our daughter, who through pregnancy was deemed "incompatible with life" by the medical professionals, who it was suggested we abort, is as I type, laying here next to me in her crib, snoring away, with no monitors, no machines and no oxygen support. She isn't just surviving, she is thriving!

GETTING TO KNOW ME

Back in February 2020, I was ready to give up, I was done with this whole life thing, I was sick of waking up every day and wishing that I hadn't. I did not want to be on this earth anymore.

The year leading up to this my life saw some massive changes, some that I wanted and I had craved for a long time, others that made me lose myself and one that saw the passing of someone very dear to me. I didn't know who I was anymore, the once strong and very capable woman, mother and business owner, turned into a weak incapable mess. Thankfully I still had my children, though I may not of been a very good mother that year, I was still a mother, and ultimately that is what saved me… that and a very special man who was about to change my life forever.

I'm Deborah – Debs, Mum to Aubrey 14, Tallulla 13 and Roux 11, all from a previous marriage, and now also Mummy to our very precious but strong, beautiful baby daughter, Jovie. Jovie's Daddy is Chris, the love of my life, the strong one, the one that pulls me up when I am down and also Dad to Cort 16, Demi-Lee 15, Sophia 12 and Keane 8. Together we make one crazy, massive, chaotic blended family and we love it!

Chris and I met about fifteen years ago when I did a family photo shoot for him, his then girlfriend and little Cort. We met like this on a few occasions as his family grew, but thought nothing of it, he was just another customer, one who I thought was punching well above his weight with such a stunning girlfriend! Fast forward fifteen years, I was out on a very rare occasion, in a pub which is somewhere you would never normally find me, but there I was after a few too many drinks talking to Chris and his friend. His friend was another previous customer of mine who I knew of more so than I did Chris. Chris and I were both in a relationship at the time, we chatted over a drink and that was it, I didn't think anymore of it.

About five months later in February 2020, up pops a friend request on my social media. I recognised the face but couldn't quite place it. Now, I'm not into accepting any strange requests, especially from men and especially after the year I had had trying to get rid of one! But as I recognised him I thought I would drop him a little message to see who he was, it read;
"Got a friend request from you… sorry not sure I know you".
And the rest, as they say, is history!

The afternoon of Wednesday 26th February was our first date, though at the time I assured him it wasn't a date at all as I was off men, for life! It was so easy, conversation just flowed, we shared secrets of our dodgy tattoos and our love for Irish men (that's another story). We of course talked about our children and Chris even joked if we were to ever have a child together it would be called "Jovi" after the band Bon Jovi. But this was our first *not* date and we already had seven children between us and we were both sure we did not want any more, so why we were talking of a child together I have no idea. Most people would run for the hills if this was mentioned on a first *not* date, but not us, the early evening ended with a kiss, two weeks later Chris had moved in!

We both soon realised that what we had, was what we

had both always been searching for. A relationship so easy, so open, so honest and with someone who was also a best friend. Not many people can say a life with seven children is easy, but ours really was, full of so much love, laughter and plenty of chaos.

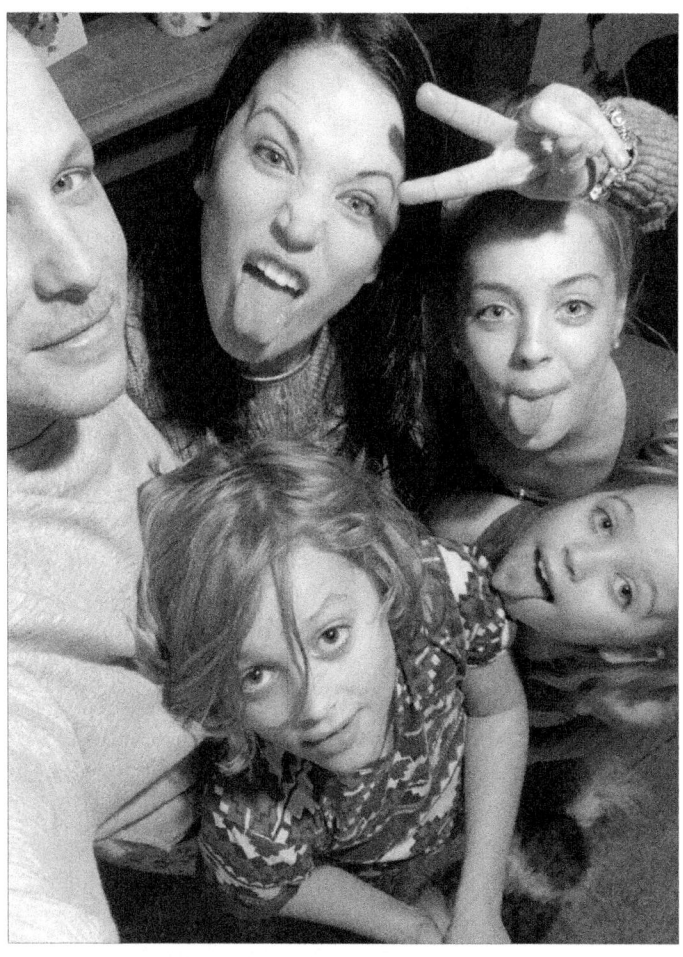

BABY MAKING

Who were we trying to kid? No more babies? How could we not, when we had finally found the kind of love we had been searching for our whole life? How could we have shared the incredible gift of bringing a baby into the world with someone else, but not each other?

Despite already having seven amazing children, we soon realised that we wanted a baby together, part of Chris and part of me. We wanted to share this love for each other with another little human, our human. Some may say that this was all a bit quick, but we knew what we felt in our hearts and that all the mistakes and lessons we had learnt in life so far were to bring us to this point. Plus, we were both pushing 35, and thought if we were to do it, we wanted to do it sooner rather than later.

Before baby making began we had a very important conversation, one that in an ideal world I think everyone should have before committing to the massive decision of making a baby. We wanted to make sure that we were both on the same page with our morals and beliefs that came with bringing a baby into this world. We already knew how each other liked to bring up children, after all we were already living that life, but we felt it important to talk about the other details. What other details you may think? I know it wouldn't even cross some people's mind that something can go wrong during pregnancy, most people expect to have a "normal" healthy baby, after all why wouldn't you think that? Maybe we did because we were older, from age 35 onwards you are at higher risk of having a baby with Down Syndrome, maybe it's because I was brought up around children with disabilities so was more aware of them, or more likely, I know it was because I was not willing to compromise my beliefs should such a situation occur. Thankfully Chris thought the same way. What I didn't know then was how important that conversation was to be.

At the end of April 2020 I came off the pill and prior to this started to take the recommended vitamins and folic acid. We were just going to see what happened and not stress too much about it. But this is me! The most impatient, needing to control, wants everything now, kind of woman! So of course I instantly downloaded a "trying to conceive" app and tracked everything. Despite having done the whole trying for a baby thing a few times before, this time was different. This time the need and excitement for this baby was equal with my partner, this time I didn't just want a baby, I wanted Chris' baby. Never in a million years did I think I would have another baby and I was so excited that it could possibly happen. I decided, because this really was going to be my last baby and a baby I never thought I would have, that I would document everything; photos, personal vlogs, symptoms – I was on it!

A month of trying and thinking I was feeling every pregnancy symptom ever; tired, bloated, sore boobs – to only then get my period! So, being ever the impatient one, out came the ovulation tests… nothing like just seeing what happened!

A month or two more of feeling every *not* pregnant pregnancy symptom, pointless ovulation tests during my still irregular cycle, a bunch of tested too early; cheapy negative pregnancy tests and of course driving Chris absolutely potty telling him when we needed to have optimum sex… we were actually, maybe, quite possibly, pregnant! It was Thursday 30th July, two days before my period was due, and despite promising myself that there would be no early testing that month, there I found myself dipping my first morning wee. Three minutes later through squinty eyes, I was adamant I saw a super faint line appear on my cheap, pound shop test strip. Flashing it in front of Chris' face at 4.30am in the morning as he was trying to leave for work, trying to make up an excuse as to why I tested early when I said I wouldn't, asking "can you see it, can you see it?" Chris really wasn't having any of it and said he wouldn't believe anything we had to squint so hard at to see. Point taken!

What seemed like the longest 24 hours of my life until I could have another first morning wee, passed by so slowly. But, just like the day before, though this time Chris was fully on board with the test, we sat waiting next to our pot of pee with a flimsy thin pregnancy test in hand, waiting our three minutes. Not having to squint *quite* so hard as the day before to see what was definitely a second line. We were pregnant! This was it, we were having a baby, our baby, my baby, his baby, made with the man I love so much.

POLAND

2020, the year the Corona Virus spread across the UK, national lockdowns and a worldwide pandemic. Only a couple of weeks after Chris and I got together, the country was forced into isolation, this is the reason Chris moved in so quickly. Even though he had only been in my life a couple of weeks, I couldn't bear the thought of not knowing how long it would be until I got to see him again, so it was pretty much all or nothing. We went for all – and we have never looked back.

Being in lockdown, in a small three bed mid-terraced house, two dogs, three children with at times six, was certainly one way to blend two separate families! It was total beautiful chaos. Mine and Chris' children all got on so well together and we filled our time with beach walks, muddy woodland hikes, out of tune karaoke and movie nights in the garden. And with Chris still working throughout the pandemic it meant I got to spend a lot of quality time alone with his children too. A lot of people hated lockdown, but having all of my favourite people under one roof, with all the time in the world, was my type of bliss. As much as I enjoyed our time in lockdown, it did mean Chris and I didn't get to go on many more dates past our first one. And even now with having Jovie, that is something that hasn't changed, but our new found trio dates are extra special.

With the talk of the first lockdown lifting and knowing we had a baby on the way, we thought we would try and squeeze in a lovely romantic weekend away. Chris was obsessed with Poland (and the blonde Polish girls!) and was desperate to take me there so I could fall in love with it too (though I didn't hear any talk of nice Polish men!) We booked it for the weekend before my birthday and just kept everything crossed that the current restrictions would still allow us to go.

Friday 14th August 2020 – I was so excited to be going away with my dream man and our tiny baby growing inside of me. I was about six or seven weeks pregnant by then, was suffering with morning sickness and already had a little bump, obviously it was more down to bloating at that stage but I loved that I could tell he or she was in there. We were still keeping the pregnancy to ourselves at this point, and I loved that only we knew.

With lockdown and a rubbish year prior, I had turned into quite an anxious person which was not really like me at all. So the thought of going on an aeroplane was a bit overwhelming, especially when I found out Chris and I weren't sitting together. However, he was the perfect gentleman and looked after me right until the last minute he could.

We touched down in the city of Krakow and it was perfect from the first breath of warm air. We had booked a lovely hotel which we got to by walking along the Vistula River, where over the weekend, we also found ourselves dining on a river boat and going kayaking. Also very popular along the river were electric scooters that you could hire. Everyone seemed to be doing it and they looked great fun so we didn't want to miss out. After seeing loads of people doubling up on one scooter, we figured we would do that too. Chris took the handlebars and I held on for dear life behind him. It really was like a romantic movie, my hands round his waist, the wind in our hair, laughing and joking the whole time. That was until; Chris hit a little bump in the road. I have honestly never laughed and nearly cried so much all at the same time. We had to keep our brave faces on and laugh through it, one because it really was hilarious but two because too many people saw us do it. We literally went over the handlebars and ended up in a heap on the floor – not the wisest move when you have a baby in tow, I know!

We continued making unforgettable memories in Krakow; trying Polish cuisine, visiting the salt mines, climbing the castle (where I was secretly hoping Chris would propose – but he didn't), dancing in a freak storm where the downpour made us wet through to our undies and securing a love lock on the bridge with our names, the children's names and of course "bump"! We had the best time, and it will remain one of our earliest memories we shared with our baby, little did we know then, how precious these memories were going to become.

AN EVENING WITH A CLAIREVOYANT

Having been back on home ground for a couple of weeks and with the children at their other parents' houses, I seized the moment to book an evening with a Clairvoyant. It was an open event with dinner all in the ticket price, meaning there were lots of other people there. I absolutely love that kind of thing and find it really brings me comfort, especially since I had lost someone very close to me the year before. It wasn't so much Chris' cup of tea, but he was happy to come along for a night out.

When booking these kind of events I am very careful not to give any personal details away as I want to make sure there is no doubt in what I get told by the Clairvoyant, should any spirits choose to come through for me. With myself and Chris still being the only ones who knew I was pregnant and wanting to make sure we kept it that way, I made sure I wore a slightly baggy top, just in case my bloated tummy looked too much like a pregnancy bump. I was only about nine weeks pregnant anyway and you really couldn't tell.

We sat patiently listening to other people's passed friends and relatives coming through to speak to them. You are never guaranteed anyone will come through for you, but either way it's still a great experience and lovely to see other people gaining comfort from the thought that their loved ones are close by. But then our time came, he looked our way, and said something along the lines of "you two are expecting a baby aren't you... only early days though", I was lost for words! He went on to tell us it was a girl. I was shocked and managed to mumble something about no one even knowing yet.

Then I asked something that I will always remember "Is everything ok though, yea?" To which he replied something or other to fob me off and continued the evening with someone else. I don't remember thinking too much of it at the time, but it's something I think a lot about now. I am certain he could sense something was wrong but I guess they don't always tell you the bad stuff. I didn't need him to tell me anyway, my mummy instinct told me very early on that something was wrong with our baby. It is that mummy instinct that I have since relied on so heavily to keep Jovie safe and well.

After that night, seeing as it was no longer just our secret, we decided it was time to tell the children.

THE ANNOUNCEMENT

I knew from the beginning of our pregnancy that I wanted to mark every occasion and create memories throughout it, at the time I put this down to it being my last pregnancy and not one I thought I would have, but subconsciously I think I just knew. The pregnancy announcement was one of those occasions I wanted to mark and make sure it was perfect.

Being a photographer, it wasn't anything unusual for me to ask the children to all come together for a photo shoot. When I handed them a t-shirt of a different colour of the rainbow for each of them to wear, maybe they thought I was a little crazy – they were "cool" almost teens / teenagers after all, but they still just got on with it and off we went to our favourite woods, my chosen location for the shoot. My idea was to take a series of photos, starting from the eldest child and adding in a child with each shot, thus building up the rainbow. Once all of the children were added in, the camera got put on timer mode and Chris and I joined the end of the rainbow, where we pulled out a crisp white baby vest with its own complete rainbow on! The children suddenly realised what this had all been about and jumped up and down with excitement. I think the announcement was a success!

Back home I edited all the photos into a short video with the caption "Fate made us the umbrella to each other's rain, together we made the sun come shining through again, and now we all wanted to let you know, that our love for each other has brightened our rainbow… Baby Manning due April 2021". (The video clip is floating around You Tube somewhere if you wanted to see it for yourself). We forwarded the video to our parents and just a select few family and friends; after all we still hadn't reached what we thought would be the safety of the twelve week mark.

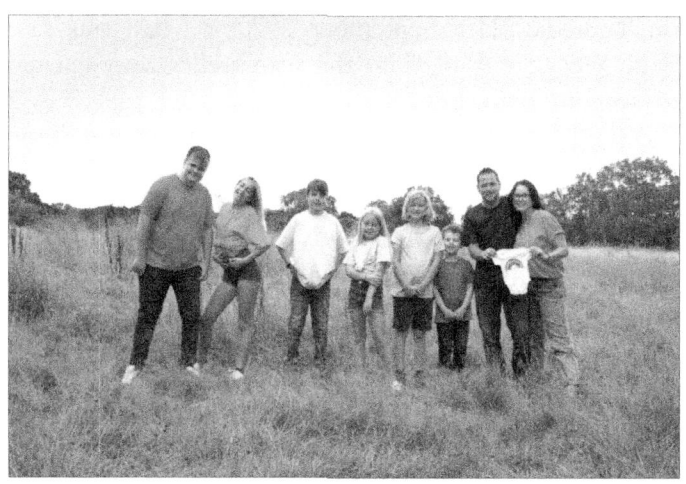

OUR TWELVE WEEK SCAN

Exactly seven months on from the day of our first *not* date and we were twelve weeks pregnant. Two days later on Thursday 24th September 2020, we had our first scan. We were going into the scan feeling very excited to see our baby but also feeling extremely nervous. I had shed lots of tears leading up to this point, call it my mummy instinct again, but I just knew something wasn't right with our baby and I feared the worst.

Laying on the bed with the cold jelly on my tummy, the sonographer started to move the doppler around. Almost instantly we saw a little heart flickering away. The relief that flooded over me was so intense, I remember looking at Chris as we gave each other a reassuring squeeze of the hand. However, it was short lived. A sense of uncertainness spread over the sonographer's face as she seemed to scan the same bit over and over again before calling for another sonographer for a second opinion. The worrying silence was finally broken with "I'm really sorry but your baby doesn't have a face." Confused, I thought to myself how can our baby not have a face? In complete disbelief I sat shocked and in silence with tears rolling down my cheeks. Whilst Chris asked all the right questions, which frustratingly she didn't have any answers to. She explained that our baby had no facial profile and was missing its nasal and maxilla bones. Her delivery of the news to us was horrendous, I will never forget her lack of empathy and this has left a deep set anxiety within me about that hospital. It already wasn't my most favourite place after a bad experience there with the birth of my first child.

Unfortunately there were no doctors available to speak to us that day and we were ushered into a private room where I sobbed uncontrollably waiting for a midwife to come and see us. When she arrived she just kept repeating the words "I'm ever so sorry" with a look of pity on her face. I wanted to scream at her "What are you sorry for? What is wrong with our baby?" questions no one was brave enough to answer. However, she did tell us our baby measured fine, and the dates were two days before what we thought so we were eleven weeks and six days pregnant, which gave us a due date of 9th April 2021. We were sent away and told to wait for a call from the bigger city hospital with a date for another appointment, this time with a fetal medicine specialist.

That evening was strange, finding comfort in each other but not in much else. Google started to become my worst enemy as I searched the words listed in our scan report and found things that I wish I hadn't. The next day was Friday, we both had to go to work which was hard but also a welcome distraction. We were still waiting for a call, one of which I received in the morning and sounded like we would have to wait a whole week to be seen. Thankfully, an afternoon call gave us an appointment for the upcoming Monday, which to me still seemed like an eternity away. The midwife on the phone advised us what would happen at the appointment and told us about the CVS screening and amniocentesis. CVS screening, Chorionic Villus Sampling, is a prenatal test used to detect birth defects, genetic diseases and other problems during pregnancy. A needle is placed in through the mother's belly right into the placenta to gather a sample of cells, and comes with a chance of miscarriage. When we told her we wouldn't be having any testing, especially the one that carried a risk to our baby's life, she sounded very shocked. But because of that conversation Chris and I had before trying for a baby, we knew neither of us were willing to compromise our baby's life for anything, this was the first time we realised our morals and beliefs sadly weren't necessarily the norm.

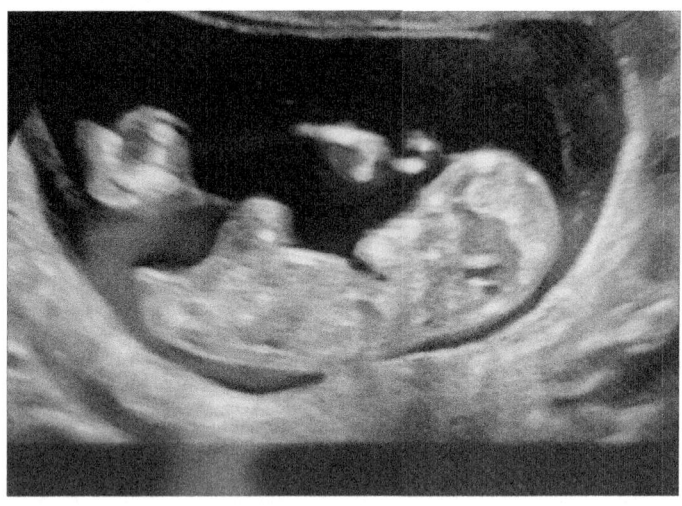

FETAL MEDICINE

After what had felt like the longest weekend ever, with barely any sleep and many, many tears, it was Monday 28th September 2020 and we were finally on our way to the city hospital. We had no idea what to expect and what they were going to tell us was wrong with our baby. Would our baby even still have a heartbeat?

It was a strange set up at the hospital. There was only one waiting room, so we were sat amongst all the excited new parents waiting to see their baby on screen for the first or maybe second time, just like we were four days prior. They would be called up for their appointment and ten minutes later come out with smiles on their faces clutching at a beautiful scan photo, just like we were supposed to. I was happy for them but I could feel the tears filling my eyes, knowing our story had started so differently.

There was a long wait for our appointment as they were running late which built up our anxiety even more. When we were eventually called in we were greeted by a lovely midwife named Rachel and a fetal medicine specialist called Alistair. Immediately we sensed they had a better bedside manner than the last sonographer did - maybe it was going to be ok? Rachel sat at the computer and Alistair began the scan, he explained he would be mumbling things to Rachel throughout but would explain his findings to us at the end. I liked them both already. Chris and I nervously gripped each other's hands, looking from the screen to each other, to Alistair, searching for some reassurance.

The scan was finished. Our baby was still alive which

was the biggest relief, but what was wrong and did our baby have a face? Though it seemed it was likely to look a little different to anyone else's, our baby did have a face! Like the other scan had shown our baby was presenting with no nasal bone and a rounder skull than usual, markers for Down Syndrome Alistair explained. Down Syndrome! Awesome! Fantastic! I understood Down Syndrome, we could handle that, I had been lucky enough to meet loads of incredible people with Down Syndrome throughout my life. Relief!... But maybe not... He then started talking about more unfamiliar conditions that I had heard of but didn't really know anything about. Alistair felt it was looking more like possible Edwards or Pataus Syndrome, these are much more serious he explained and not all babies with these conditions make it to term. It was all a bit of a blur, I'm not really sure how the whole conversation went but we did discuss what options were open to us. He said we could have the routine nuchal test which consisted of bloods from me and a scan of the baby's neck. We had originally said we didn't want these, after all no matter what was wrong with our baby we knew what we would or more to the point, wouldn't do. Though, as this was non-invasive we were now considering it, however Alistair explained that his findings from the scan he had just done showed the fluid on the back of the neck actually looked in a good range anyway. The other option was a CVS test now and / or an amniocentesis later on in the pregnancy. These were invasive procedures and carried a risk to our baby, so they weren't an option for us. After we had refused the invasive tests, I think Alistair knew the answer to his next question was pretty obvious, but we understood he had to make all the options clear to us. Despite not having any further tests to confirm, our scan was conclusive enough for him to offer us a termination on medical grounds. We didn't even hesitate with our refusal, we knew this was never an option for us. Our baby had a heartbeat and so long as its heart was beating we would let him or her tell their own story.

ONLY DOWN SYNDROME

It was seven weeks and three days until we got to see our baby again. That's 52 days we were left to process this information, or lack of, that we had been given, and 52 days of wondering if our baby was even still alive. I reverted to my usual way of coping - Google, even though I knew most of the time it only filled me with more fear. Though, my search made me stumble across a group called "PADS – Positive About Down Syndrome" which was started by a Mum whose son has Down Syndrome. Other parents who were pregnant with a definite Down Syndrome diagnosis would post on this group seeking positivity from others living with the diagnosis. I read through them all, the upset and the tears about their baby having Down Syndrome and I could only think how lucky they were that they *only* had a Down Syndrome diagnosis. How I longed to know that my baby *only* had Down Syndrome. Writing this, I'm under no illusion that I sound pretty awful saying *only* Down Syndrome, I know I sound like I am not validating anyone else's fears and the reality of living with this diagnosis, and I know that in worst cases Down Syndrome or what comes with it can still be fatal. But I understood Down Syndrome, I had heard of it, I knew what it was, I fully believed all these amazing positive stories on the group from other parents who felt blessed to have been given a child with Down Syndrome, because throughout my life I had these positive experiences myself too. The truth is, after our scan I knew something was seriously wrong with our baby and for it to have *only* Down Syndrome would have been our best possible chance at having a life with our baby in it, it meant we could still have hope.

It was a long seven weeks where we tried so hard to remain positive and make as many memories as possible with our unborn baby inside of me. We took lots of photos of my growing bump, a bump that was no longer easy to hide. Part of me didn't want to hide it, I wanted to savour every second of the pregnancy and for people to know my baby existed and was growing. But then surely people would congratulate us and we wouldn't know what to say. Did we just say thank you and move on or tell them that our baby wasn't like everyone else's?

The next scan date was getting closer, I thought I had been feeling the odd flutter from the baby and my bump was growing, so I still remained hopeful that everything would be ok. The life we imagined we would have with our baby might have changed but at least there would still be a life. Right? We managed to almost convince ourselves that we would be one of the lucky parents blessed with a baby rocking an extra Chromosome 21. It would all be ok.

THE NEXT SCAN

It was 19th November 2020, Covid-19 (Corona Virus) was still very much taking hold of the world but the children had at least returned to school, though any type of cough and they were being sent home. Typically this day, our son Roux, had a cough. Normally it wouldn't have been a problem but we were about to go to the hospital for our long awaited next scan. Not an ideal situation but we had no choice than to take him in the car with us.

52 days since our last scan, now 19 weeks and six days pregnant, and we were back at the city hospital sitting in a waiting room anxiously waiting to see and hear the fate of our unborn child. The thoughts in our mind flitting between was our baby even still alive, to it all being a mistake and our baby was perfectly fine, wanting to get in the room and see our baby, to not wanting to go in there so we didn't have to hear any more bad news. Then remembering whatever they told us we were going to have to go straight out and face our 11 year old son who was waiting in the car. As anxious as we were though, I really think the stronger feeling we had was that it was all going to be ok.

I climbed onto the bed, gripping Chris' hand as tightly as he could allow, pulled up my top to reveal my baby bump that had still been growing, tucked the tissue into the waistband on my trousers and waited for the squirt of cold gel. Our baby soon appeared on the screen followed by its little flickering heart. Our baby was still alive! Those flutters I thought I had been feeling really were our baby. Same as before, the doctor starts moving the doppler around, mumbling to the midwife in the room, reassuring us he would explain everything to us once he had finished. I looked at Chris, Chris looked at me, we both looked at the doctor just trying to get something, anything from his facial expressions. Was our baby ok? "I'm sorry to report some serious abnormalities in the fetus" he pronounced. What we had pinned our hopes on, Down Syndrome, couldn't have been further from the truth. The doctor pulled his chair closer to us, leant forward resting his arms onto his knees and in his soft Irish accent told us "the brain is abnormal, the appearance suggests Alobar Holoprosencephaly" it was worse than any of us thought. He still didn't rule out Edwards or Patau's Syndrome, but made it pretty clear that regardless of the genetic condition, the brain condition alone was likely to be fatal.

Once again we were advised of all the options, and told that we could choose to terminate our baby right up until full term due the extent of the medical condition it had. What was I hearing? I had a big noticeable baby bump, I could feel my baby move, yet we could decide to kill it whilst its heart was still beating? And at this point, through choice, I still hadn't even had any tests other than the normal scans, but yet they were still so sure. Our heads were a mess but termination was never for us and we quickly dismissed that option. Again, we were also informed about an amniocentesis, which could have been done there and then. It is something we considered in the moment, despite always thinking we wouldn't have this done, but we just didn't know what to do for the best. Then I remembered that our son was still waiting in the car and we had already been much longer than we had told him we would be. I felt so conflicted, I just couldn't make any decisions.

Thankfully the midwife and the doctor were both amazing and told us there was absolutely no reason to make any decisions in that moment. They booked us in for another scan for a week later and referred us to Great Ormond Street Hospital for an in depth scan of our baby's heart, due to a possible associated cardiac defect. We wiped our tears, took a deep breath and found our brave faces for the car journey home.

GENDER REVEAL

Most parents go to their 20 week scan and find out the gender of their baby, not be told it's likely they won't even get to meet their baby alive. Before our previous scan we had decided we weren't going to find out if we were having a boy or a girl and when they offered to tell us we declined. But in the week that followed after the devastating news that our baby was likely to pass, we decided we wanted to find out after all. We wanted to be able to call them our "son" or our "daughter" for as long as possible and we still wanted to celebrate the life that we had created and that was growing inside of me. We had a week to wait until we could find out if we were having a boy or a girl. Either way, as you know, it was always going to be named Jovi.

Just four days after our referral we were on our way to Great Ormond Street Hospital, about three to four hours away from our home. We drove most of the way there and then parked up to catch a tube into the city. Chris doesn't drive, only rides a motorbike, and even though I am a very confident driver I did not like the idea of driving into London and finding somewhere to park. I wouldn't want to do this in any situation, let alone one that was already very stressful.

The hospital seemed nice and welcoming with helpful volunteers showing us where we were supposed to be going. Chris was allowed into the waiting room with me but due to Covid-19 restrictions (bloody Covid!) he was not allowed into the scan room. I was petrified to be on my own and listen to any more bad news they may have to tell me, plus my hearing is not the best and I was worried I would miss something important. Thankfully it all went well, they think there may have been a small hole in the heart but nothing that made them concerned. Finally, a bit of good news!

26th November 2020, a week on since we received the devastating blow that our baby had Alobar Holoprosencephaly, and we were back at the city hospital, thankfully without a child waiting in the car for us! During our scan we asked the question whether a definite chromosomal diagnosis would make any difference to the care of our baby and received the answer that it wouldn't. We were told an amniocentesis carried a risk of miscarriage to one in 100 fetuses, this may seem fairly minimal to some but when we were already pregnant with a one in 16,000 baby, one in 100 seemed way too risky. So due to the risk and the fact it would make no difference to the care our baby would receive we stuck to our original thoughts and decided against any invasive testing. The odds were already stacked against us and we did not want to lessen our chances even more. So this turned out to be just another scan, to repeat all the bad news and to add to the what seemed like an ever growing list of medical problems. We learnt our baby also had Microcephaly. Despite this, there was still an element of excitement at this scan as we asked them to look at the gender of our baby. But to change it up a bit we kindly asked them not to disclose the gender to us and instead to write it down and put it in a sealed envelope. We were going to have a gender reveal!

Driving home knowing we had the gender of our baby in our hands was almost too much to bear, I nearly started to regret the idea of a gender reveal as I just wanted to know what we were having there and then.

We had decided we would reveal it with a cake, so we drove the envelope straight to a friend of mine who is a professional cake maker and left it all in her capable hands, with the only specification of the cake being elephant themed.

With us still being at the height of Covid we were limited as to what we could do for the gender reveal. We decided on a Facebook live reveal so invited everyone to join us virtually just two days after the gender had been hidden in the envelope. We had all the children at home and decorated the house with pink and blue balloons, I wanted to make sure it was a moment to remember. Prior to the reveal, Chris, myself and all the children wrote down our guesses as to whether we thought we were having a boy or a girl. Up to this point in pregnancy I was adamant we were having a girl, but I think Chris got inside my head and made me think it was a boy. I know Chris would have loved to have a little boy, he wanted a little him running around charming all the ladies! But neither of us really minded, all we wished for was that our baby got to take a breath on the outside world.

With the camera on the tripod, the laptop ready to go and the cake taking pride of place in the middle of the room, we went live on Facebook. The cake was a beautiful two tiered cake with an elephant topper. I did a little speech at the start whilst nervously waving around a big cake knife, where I had to stop myself from crying when I mentioned how extra special this baby was to us. We were soon cutting into the cake with everyone eagerly watching what colour sponge we would reveal inside the cake, "It's pink, it's pink" Roux shouts, before I had even got the knife through the cake. Sure enough, when I cut out a slice, it was most certainly pink. We were having a girl! Our daughters were thrilled, more so because they made bets with Chris and were in to win some money from the revelation of it being a girl. If you do a You Tube search of our "Our Gender Reveal after Holoprosencephaly Diagnosis" you can hear them excitedly shouting "We get money, we get money!"

So there it was, our amazing little baby, became our daughter, Jovie (with an e!)

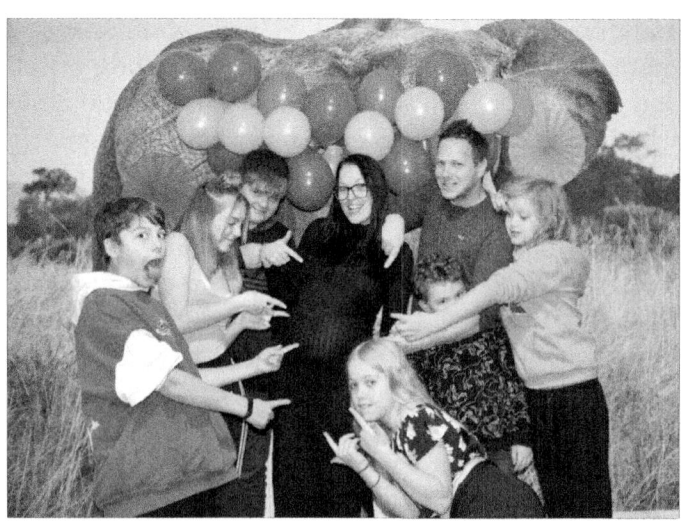

THE BEGINNING OF "JOVIE'S JOURNEY – OUR SPECIAL LITTLE GIRL"

On our first date I revealed to Chris that I was one of six siblings, which I have always thought was quite a lot. However, Chris completely outdid me when he told me he was one of fourteen! That soon shut me up. It turned out I had actually photographed quite a lot of his siblings and nephews and nieces in the past as we live in quite a small town.

With both of us having such big families we found ourselves constantly having to repeat the same bad news about Jovie's medical problems over and over, when all we really wanted to do was enjoy our daughter whilst we could and celebrate her as much as possible. This is when we decided to make a Facebook page dedicated to her and "Jovie's Journey – our special little girl" was born. The initial idea of it was just to be able to keep family and close friends in the loop about our pregnancy and for Jovie to enter their hearts like she did ours, little did we know then how much the page would grow and how far Jovie's story would spread.

Our first post on the page explained what we had been through to date in the pregnancy which was then followed by this excerpt;

…after many tears and heartbreaking conversations, we are now at a point where we just want to share and celebrate our special baby girl's life whilst we still have her.

As strong believers of "everything happens for a reason", I know we were blessed with this baby girl for a reason. However long or short her journey may be, our love for her will never falter and she is already changing our lives for the better. Whilst we move forward with hope in our heart, that a miracle may let us bring our baby girl home one day, we are realistic that our time with her in my belly may be cut short.

So we ask you to please celebrate our little girl with us as if she were already here, don't say "sorry" to us for our news, for we are not sorry that we were chosen to be the parents of this unique and special and beautiful baby girl."

This page became my therapy and writing became my coping mechanism, it soon became more than I ever planned it to be.

<u>*8th December 2020 – 22 weeks*</u>
Knowing Jovie could leave us at any time makes each movement I feel so precious, her kicks seem to be getting stronger every day, Daddy can even feel them now too. Not much sleep being had because as soon as I close my eyes, my mind goes into overdrive about what we have to come, and I just lay there willing her to move so I know she is ok, and I don't want to miss a single kick. I know our little girl is a fighter and whatever time we have together we will always be grateful for.

22 weeks of loving you and lifetime left of love to give you."

16th December 2020

My heart hurts for you baby, how I wish you didn't have to go away,
I want to cradle you in my arms, where a lifetime you can stay.
My heart hurts for you baby, when I feel you moving around,
I pray I will get to hear, your crying little sound.
My heart hurts for you baby, and the thoughts of what we could of had,
With your brothers and sisters, me and your amazing Dad.
My heart hurts for you baby, I am so trying to be strong,
But a night with the thoughts in my head, is just too long.
My heart hurts for you baby, but I am so grateful it was me,
Chosen to be your Mummy, from now to eternity.

19th December 2020

Some days it's hard to believe, that anything could be wrong,
As your wriggles and kicks are getting, so very strong.
You really like the evening, when Daddy and I lay together,
Memories we will hold in our heart, for the rest of forever.
To think the doctors told us, we could cut your life short,
This was never a choice we needed to give any thought.
For whether you are born sleeping, or if a miracle means you are born to stay,
The world can take all my tears, for what you already give me everyday.

27th December 2020

Our baby girl Jovie we spent Christmas with you,
You received gifts and were thought of, all the way through.
There still lies a present for you under the tree,
From all the big ones, your Daddy and from me.
I'm trying to keep hope that we can open it together,
And share in happy times for the rest of forever.
Christmas was hard because with hopes come fears,
That sometimes make me too overcome with tears.
But as always your Daddy was here by my side,
To hold me and kiss my head as I cried.
But we both know that even with things as they are,
Still feeling you move was our greatest Christmas gift so far.

NEW YEARS EVE

We had just enjoyed our first ever Christmas, not just together, but with our baby girl growing inside of me. It was a lovely Christmas but full of lots of different emotions. We made sure there was a present for Jovie under the tree, after all, it might be the only chance we ever get to buy her a Christmas present and it wasn't just us that bought her a gift either. My big brother, Jovie's Uncle Simon, bought her some sound books so she could hear them in the womb. Roux couldn't wait to get reading them to her.

It was now New Years Eve and we were 25 weeks and six days pregnant, it had been about five weeks since our previous scan and we were back at the city hospital waiting for another. I felt super excited we were going to get to see our baby again. That's one positive I guess we could say about all this, we certainly got to see our baby on an ultrasound more than usual and as it was a high risk pregnancy it meant Chris got to come in to all of the scans with me. Unfortunately that wasn't the case for a lot of new parents, due to the risk of Covid-19 transmission there were a lot of restrictions in place.

For this appointment and every one going forward, I started to take a bag with me, probably the hardest bag I have ever had to pack. What do you put in a bag for *just in case* your baby has died inside you and will need delivering, or *just in case* the medical team decide they need to get her out in an emergency? We got Jovie a special elephant blanket and matching taggy made, so if the worst was to happen both us and Jovie could keep something that was matching. We also packed a hand and foot casting kit to make some keepsakes with her.

There were other bits added into the bag as time went on, when I felt brave enough to buy some nappies or a special outfit. I went in many a shop to find that special outfit, and most times I just burst into tears or walked straight back out again. I was just too scared to tempt fate or to let myself get excited about buying outfits for a baby I had been told wouldn't even take a breath.

At this scan we got to see Jovie in 4d, as usual she had her hand up to her face for most of it. We always joked that having her clenched fist up proved she was ready to fight like we needed her to. This time the extent of her cleft lip was also very visible. It was made very clear to us, once again, the severity of Jovie's condition and the unlikeliness of her survival. Even though we already knew all this, it seemed really hard to take all over again, almost like the first time they told us. I had just had about five weeks since her last scan, of feeling her kicks getting nice and strong and I guess I was secretly hoping that all the bad stuff had gone away somehow. But no, I was certainly brought back down to earth with a very big dose of reality.

10th January 2021

*People keep saying something to me, but I think they are wrong
They say I'm doing really well and being really strong.
But they don't see the sleepless nights when I'm still awake at three,
Drowning in my tears, with Daddy comforting me.
They aren't in my head when you are all I can think about,
Trying to be full of hope but mainly full of doubt.
They don't feel you kick, Daddy says it's your way of saying you're ok,
Seeking any comfort I can from you, to get me through the day.
Some people say it's amazing what we have chosen to do!
But I don't get it, you're our daughter, we could never give up on you.*

Her Story To Tell

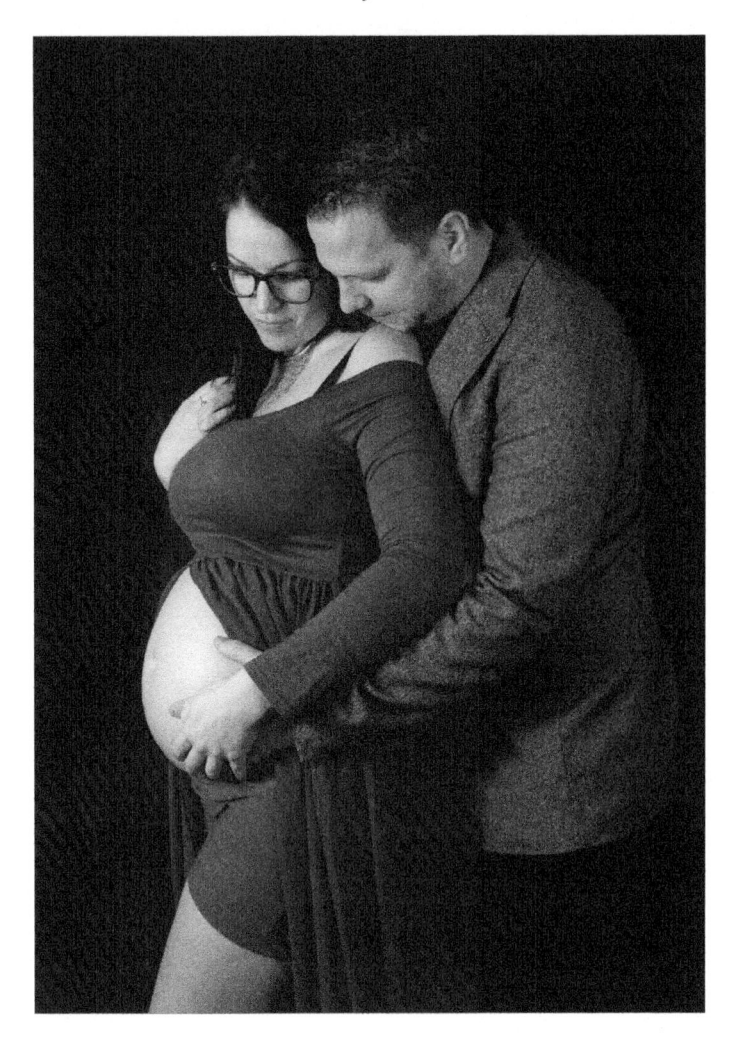

HYPNOBIRTHING

I had just turned 22 years old when I gave birth to my first son, Aubrey, in September 2007. I loved every bit of my pregnancy, despite it being unplanned and making me a single Mum, it also kind of saved me. I was at a place in my life where I was just lost, I didn't have much direction, I was holding down a full time job but out of work I was just "meh" and my mental health was really starting to suffer. Finding out I was pregnant was the kick up the butt I needed, I knew I had to look after myself and look after my baby so I booked myself in for some counselling sessions to sort out whatever was going on in my head at the time. To this day, I am still a big fan of counselling, I am not embarrassed to say I can be a head case sometimes and I need help figuring out my complicated mind every now and then. More so than ever recently!

I was so excited about my pregnancy and the idea of having a baby that I read all about how he or she was developing each week. But as far as the birth went, looking back now I really didn't give it much thought. More than a week after my due date, my contractions started and to be honest I was a bit of a wimp! I didn't cope great with them at home so off I went to the hospital, bag packed, expecting to have a baby a little while later. With no pre thought out birthing plan, I thought I would just show up at the hospital, the midwives would tell me what to do and I would have my baby. How very mistaken I was. The pain seemed unbearable but I was sent home once as labour hadn't even started! When finally allowed to stay in the hospital, I was given Pethidine and an Epidural, meaning all I then wanted to do was sleep. The most vivid memory I have of the birth experience was of my midwife, she was an older lady, dressed in her uniform but with bare legs which I don't think had ever met a shaver before because I just remember repeatedly seeing how hairy they were! She kept telling me I was lazy and I needed to wake up, yet she was the one that drugged me up with all this stuff! I'm sure she saw me as much younger than I was (I have always looked younger than my age) and she had made her opinion up about me on whatever basis she decided to do that on. None of the experience was how I thought giving birth was going to be and none of it was how I would ever want it to be again. It ended with my legs up in stirrups, my son being pulled out by ventouse and an addition of some delightful stitches down in my lady bits – oh and somewhere along the line I shit myself, put my foot in it and smeared it across the bed! Lovely!

My beautiful brown eyed boy was born, Aubrey Ronan James, weighing 8lb 15 and a half oz! I was elated to take him home and not spend a minute longer in the hospital, it just did not feel a nice safe place to be as a new mum, and I vowed I would never be giving birth there again. However, I am a strong believer that our experiences are what shape our future, and I can now thank that awful midwife for teaching me how important it is to own and take control of our own births.

Staying true to my word I never gave birth in that hospital again. For the birth of my daughter, Tallulla Hannah in 2009, weighing an amazing 10lb 4oz, and the birth of my son, Roux William Ewart in 2010, weighing an even bigger 10lb 12oz, I opted for a home birth. I thought it might be wise to do a little bit more reading about the actual birth process for those ones! I found myself reading a hypnobirthing book, it was an interesting read but I didn't channel too much time or practice into it at the time, so it didn't help me as much as it could have during my subsequent births, but I think it definitely planted a seed in my mind. Surrounded by my own home comforts, the children around me, a birthing pool in my bedroom, and no medical interventions that I knew nothing about, I had two much calmer birth experiences.

Later in 2015 I was lucky enough to experience another wonderful home birth, this time when I gave birth to my friends' baby girl, Miya. I loved my last two births so much that I decided to do it all over again but for someone else! Being a surrogate is one of my biggest achievements in life, I felt so privileged to be entrusted to carry and grow someone else's little human. Miya was biologically her Mum and Dad's, I just provided the womb in which to grow her. It was so important to me that Miya's Mum felt as included in the birth process as possible and when it was time for Miya to enter the world, her Mum joined me in the birthing pool and caught her own daughter as she was born into the water. Miya left me and went straight into the arms of her Mum, with her Dad there too. It really was the most beautiful moment and one I will remain proud of forever. But surrogacy is a whole other story and since all of our complications with Jovie our eyes have been very opened to what a horror story surrogacy could potentially turn out to be, but that is for another book!

As previously mentioned I am a professional photographer and during my pregnancy with Jovie I was at a customer's house doing her family photos. Her name is Heidi, I had done her family photos a few times before and we got on well. Heidi spoke about her own home birth experience and how she had become a hypnobirthing instructor for The Wise Hippo Birthing Programme. I let her know the medical challenges we were facing with this pregnancy. The seed that had been planted from reading that book about 14 years ago had suddenly just been watered again. Maybe hypnobirthing was what I needed to help me positively navigate the rest of this pregnancy and birth. A couple of weeks later Heidi contacted me saying she would like to gift me her hypnobirthing teaching programme, I was absolutely overwhelmed with her kindness. Not quite knowing at the time the full extent to which it would help me, to now shouting from the roof tops about how amazing it is.

This act of kindness from Heidi was the first in a long line that we slowly started to notice throughout our journey with Jovie. We started realizing more and more that Jovie was given to us for a reason, and she was perfectly the way she was supposed to be, our child was changing people and was teaching kindness and empathy before she had even entered the world.

Our sessions with Heidi began, Chris was a bit sceptical about it all at first but was happy to take part as he knew it was what I wanted. He also quickly learnt that there were a lot of opportunities where he could fall asleep during the hypnotic music practice! Heidi taught us not only how to have a pain free birth but how to take control of our birth, how to ask the right questions and empowered us to feel confident in my ability to birth Jovie the way I wanted. She made me realize that regardless of what may happen with Jovie, birthing her was not an option and it was something I would have to do no matter what, so I may as well make it a positive experience with positive memories. Most people seem to think that as soon as there are medical complications with the baby or pregnancy all the say you have in your birth becomes nonexistent. Heidi taught us that this is not the case and everything was still our choice. Of course we would never ever put our baby at unnecessary risk but the medical team were going to very much have to justify their opinions to me if they wanted anything different to us. Thankfully, when we approached our fetal medicine doctor about my need to have a natural unassisted water birth, he was all for it, I couldn't quite believe my ears. In fact, he even said if I really wanted her at home like my others then he would try to accommodate that too. At that point I remember saying "Don't just try and appease me as you think she is going to die anyway". He assured me that's not what he was doing, however, even I thought a home birth was a step too crazy given the circumstances.

Hypnobirthing is all about positivity, letting go of any negatives that people so often try and associate with birth and instead focus on your perfect birth. Along with lots of positive birth affirmations, on 12th January 2021, Heidi got us to write out our perfect birth story, with the idea that it would become self fulfilling…

We are excited and organised for the day of Jovie's birth. Our bags are packed with all of our chosen special things, for our perfect birth. My parents arrive to take care of the children and the dogs. We say our goodbyes which are full of love and hugs.

Our journey to the hospital is calm, there is no traffic, and Chris has his comforting hand on my leg. I have full trust in Chris and the hospital we are on our way to, that they will take good care of myself and Jovie.

We arrive at the hospital, park easily and are warmly greeted by the staff who are expecting our arrival. We settle into our room and set up our things to make it feel as calm, relaxed and as homely as possible.

The birthing process progresses nicely and I remain free to walk around and stay as mobile as possible. I do not require any pain relief, my practice of hypnobirthing and the comfort from Chris is making the process a pleasurable and empowering experience. I have relaxing music playing, read through my birth affirmations and Chris knows exactly what to say and do to keep me focused. Jovie remains calm throughout and works in harmony with my body to progress down the birth canal, just as she should.

Throughout it all the atmosphere is calm and relaxed with lots of laughter, smiles and love. Photos and videos are being taken to capture this momentous time in our lives.

Jovie is now ready to meet her Mummy & Daddy, I breathe her out through her final journey into the world, reaching down to touch her head as she comes.

She cries. She is breathing. She is ours.

Chris is the first to touch Jovie, he gathers her and places her on my chest for skin to skin contact, and he holds us both whilst we take in this moment of being complete with our baby girl. Once Jovie's cord has stopped pulsating, Chris cuts the cord, shuffles on the bed beside me and has skin to skin cuddles with Jovie too. All the time this is happening the atmosphere is calm and relaxed with lots of photos and videos being taken.

When the time comes for the doctors to check Jovie over, they are able to do it in the room with us and communicate well throughout. We get to stay with Jovie throughout her care. Chris and I feel blessed to finally have our baby girl here with us, and take strength from having each other and having Jovie, to get us through whatever comes our way.

Our children are given the opportunity to meet their new baby sister, showering her with love, whilst lots of photos being taken and one of us all as our big happy family.

<u>*15th January 2021*</u>
Somedays it's just too much to bear,
The thought of the day when you will no longer be there.
We are 28 weeks today, and I'm grateful you are feeling strong,
But it's just another week closer, to when it could all go wrong.
You are our little girl, half of Daddy and half of me,
You turn us from being a couple, into being three.
I don't want that taken from us, I want you to stay,
I don't want there to be a time, that you get taken away.
This is the hardest thing that we have ever had to do,
Preparing for your death, before we've even got to meet you.
Staying realistic so it doesn't hit us so hard,
But hoping we get dealt that one lucky card.
No matter how much this hurts there will never be a day,
That we regret letting nature lead us the right way.
So as I lay here in the dark, all I can do is pray,
That we will get to bring our little girl home one day.

DONOR BABY

As the pregnancy continued, every day felt like another battle we had won. We still had all the usual pregnancy appointments to attend on top of our extra care ones, including the MRI scan we had previously been referred for. We had to go to a different hospital for the MRI scan, a couple of hours away from home. Chris came with me and helped me find the correct ward but then he had to go back and sit in the car due to restrictions still being in place. I was shown into a little cubicle where I was handed a hospital gown to change into and a fresh face mask (the fashion accessory of the year due to Covid-19!) I was asked to remove all of my jewellery and then was taken through for the scan. I had never had an MRI scan before and with my anxiety it wasn't a pleasant experience. It was very noisy, I felt like I was laying on the floor of an aeroplane cargo hold. Weirdly, I didn't feel worried about the results though, what more could they possibly tell us was wrong with Jovie's brain than they already had. But I was definitely glad when it was over.

Ten days later, 28th January 2021, we were back for another scan with the fetal medicine doctor at the city hospital. They ran through the MRI results with us and informed us that the scan was consistent of that of Semi-Lobar Holoprosencephaly, a little better than the original Alobar Holoprosencephaly they had diagnosed. Though he explained it made very little difference at all to the expectations they had for Jovie.

After this scan we got to meet a neo-natal doctor who was able to give us a bit more information on what choices there were for after birth. We had to start to discuss the kind of care plan we would like to follow should Jovie be born alive or if we would want them to intervene if she wasn't breathing for herself. They explained how they may be able to place a tiny tube down her throat to breath for her but they were unsure due to her facial deformities. It was a really hard conversation to be part of and I think I got through a whole box of tissues whilst doing so. But between Chris and I we had already decided that we wouldn't push Jovie too far, as hard as that decision was to make, we said that she had to show us she was up for the fight.

As well as the neo-natal doctor we also met another amazing midwife who I had requested to see about expressing breast milk. I have always been a keen breast feeder and as a former breastfeeding support worker I knew just how amazing breast milk was, especially for sick babies. It was so important to me they knew that I wanted Jovie to only have breast milk and I wanted their advice about how soon I could start expressing. The midwife was so lovely and helpful and was able to answer all of my questions. What was really special about her though was she sat in front of us and she used our baby's name as if she was already here. She cried for our baby, a baby she hadn't even met yet but who had really touched her heart. She told us how she admired our strength and determination to give our baby a chance. I will never forget this midwife. Strong is often a word people used to describe us, ironic really as mentally I felt like I was crumbling.

The final person we met that day was Natalie, a donor nurse. Even though she was wearing a face mask you could just tell she had a lovely kind face, I liked her immediately and like the midwife, our story really touched Natalie. Once again, this was a special request of ours for her to come and speak to us. It was always a no brainer for us, if Jovie wasn't able to stay Earth side herself then we hoped she could save another baby's life instead. We always knew Jovie had a purpose and it was up to us to explore each avenue so she had the opportunity to fulfil that purpose. We learnt that despite whatever chromosome abnormality Jovie had she could still be a donor. I felt so relieved and so proud that my little girl could do something so amazing.

29th January 2021
They called you by your name today it was really nice to hear,
The midwife when she spoke of you even shed a tear.
Already you are touching so many lives on earth,
Imagine your great impact by the time of your coming birth.
I know you were sent to us to teach the world so much,
And already you are doing that without a single touch.
This world will learn one day to see the beauty in what we are blessed,
And not filter out the ones that don't conform with all the rest.
Together you and I, can get their fog to lift,
And teach them all that every life, is the greatest ever gift.

KEEPING A GOOD BALANCE

On our first date, Chris and I discovered we were alike in so many ways, but as our relationship developed we discovered we were also very different. It has been these differences that has really helped us get through this journey together.

I am a worrier. I think of everything that could possibly happen before it happens. I like to be organised and prepare for every eventuality. I think of all the what ifs. I Google, I search and I arm myself with as much information as possible. I can never switch off. My sleep is haunted by my daytime thoughts. And I cry, a lot. Chris however, is none of the above! He is super positive, always finds the good in a negative situation, goes with the flow, doesn't have any need for advanced organization and just rolls with the day. Unlike me, Chris avoided Google like the plague and kept the mentality that, whilst our baby had a heartbeat then we should enjoy every moment and not let the time we had with our baby growing, be spoilt by what might happen. And crying is something he doesn't often do, in fact, never. We have learnt that to get through this journey we need both of our ways and need to learn from each other's traits. Not one way is right and not one way is enough, life requires a balance to keep our head above water and keep moving forward.

So many times through pregnancy I have thought back to that fall we had in Poland, I have wondered if it was our fault and whether we were the ones that caused Jovie's medical condition. Hundreds of google searches later and I know it wasn't us, I know she was just a tiny little dot fully protected inside of me and I know what is wrong with Jovie is a chromosomal abnormality and "just one of those things". But, the first thing you do with such news like we got in pregnancy, is to blame yourself. Nowadays though we look back and laugh, have a bit of a private joke about the scooter incident, which some might say is a little tasteless given the circumstances, but one thing we have learnt is we still have to laugh.

We tried to balance out the turmoil of our pregnancy with lots of fun happy memories whenever we could. On 8th February 2021, it snowed, it really properly snowed. It was so white and crisp and so beautiful. With the ground covered in a blanket of what looked like fluffy clouds, it was too perfect of a photo opportunity to miss! I put on my long purple maternity dress, it had long sleeves with a sheer opening at the front, which lightly brushed my bare pregnancy bump, showing it to the fresh cold air. With some black leggings on and a grey wooly hat, my daughter Tallulla and I headed out into the snow. Tallulla took charge of the camera and I started to play in the snow as if Jovie were there with us. It was a bitter sweet moment as I knew it was likely to be the only opportunity I got to share the snow with her. I sprinkled the snow on my belly so she could feel how cold it was.

8th February 2021

To our little Jovie Jean, snow lays upon the ground,
It's settled on the rooftops and is laying all around.
It allows my mind to dream, of when you see it too,
Maybe this time next year, when we've had a whole year with you?
We will wrap you up warm and take you out into the snow,
At your Daddy and me, a snowball you could throw.
You can feel the snow crunch and how cold it is to touch,
Never a dream, have I wanted so much.
For now it makes me smile and a dream it will stay,
But if the time ever comes, it will be the best ever day!

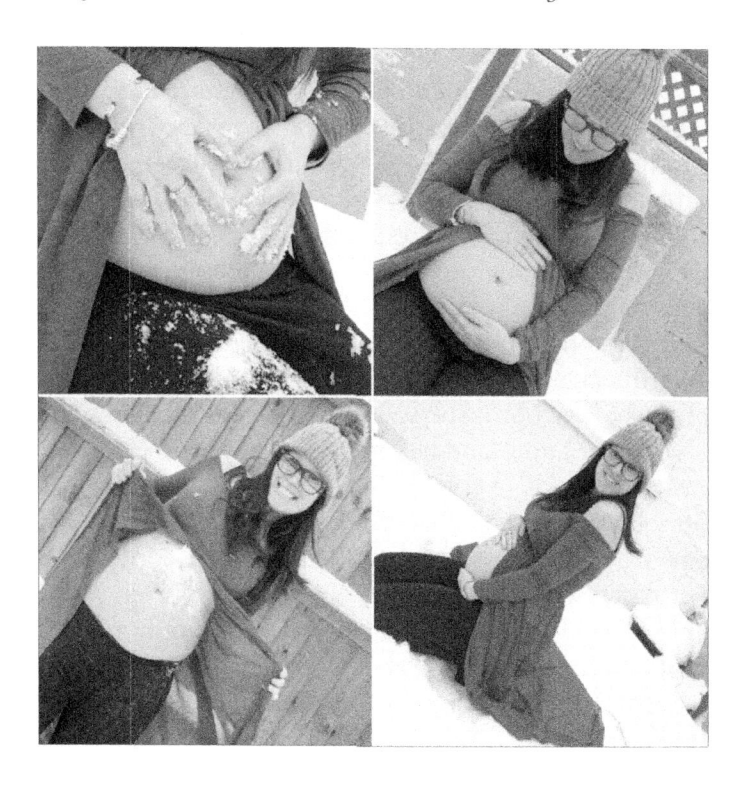

I was now reaching the 33 week milestone, a milestone that only a couple of months before felt so unattainable. One thing this pregnancy was teaching me was gratitude, pure and utter thankfulness for every second our baby girl was giving us. I would constantly be learning of success stories from parents who had gone on the same "incompatible with life" journey as us, seeing their child hit a first, tenth or even an eighteenth birthday! My hope would grow that maybe, just maybe, we could be one of those success stories too. But then as frequently as I heard of a success story I would learn of another baby or child whose life had been cut short and it would hit me like another big slap in the face.

It was during this time in my pregnancy that I learnt of Aurora. Aurora was part of a twin pregnancy with her brother Oliver. Aurora was also diagnosed with Alobar Holoprosencephaly, the same as Jovie. Aurora is daughter to Rob and Crystal, from across the globe to us, but even though so far in distance our journeys were so similar. I only learnt of Aurora just after she was born, through her Facebook page similar to Jovie's. Heartbreakingly Aurora passed away just eleven days after she was born, she was at home surrounded by the love of her family and her gorgeous baby brother.

So selflessly, Rob and Crystal shared her with the world and I for one are so grateful that they did. Along with her parents, she has shaped my journey massively and I am so grateful I got to know of her and I am honoured to now call Rob and Crystal my friends. This is when I realized, I was allowing "success" stories to be rated by the number of birthdays that were celebrated or milestones that were met. When the truth is, all of these fetuses, babies and children are success stories from the moment they are conceived. They each have their own story to tell, and however long they are given in the womb or on earth, they are given to us to teach love, gratitude, empathy, kindness, friendship, understanding and so many life lessons we may not otherwise experience. I certainly know that I took my other pregnancies for granted, it's only when you are faced with the fear of it being taken away do you truly understand gratitude.

<u>12th February 2021</u>
Over 40,000 people ran in the London Marathon. When they entered the marathon how many of them do you think actually believed that they had a chance at coming first place in the race? 100? 500? Certainly no where near all of them! I'm sure some of them even doubted whether they would cross the finish line at all!

So why did they enter? They entered for all the amazing feelings and memories they would gain from the experience. Whatever place they crossed the line at, if they crossed it at all, no one could take those things away from them, and they would certainly be finishing the race a more fulfilled person than what they started.

Imagine if you were standing on that start line, after months of training, ready to run that marathon, and then you look down and realize your laces are undone. Do you give up, leave them undone and say you can't run? Or do you retie them and start that race?
To us, termination was like giving up and leaving our laces undone.
If we had done that, we would have missed out on so much, we would never have got to feel this indescribable, unconditional love for our baby girl that really is like no other, we would never of got those moments together feeling her kick and watching her grow, we would of never known her story, we would of never connected

together as a couple in a way that is stronger and deeper than ever imaginable, we would never of discovered this empathy for others and this gratitude for life we now have.

Like any marathon it has had its high points and low points, but together they have created the most unforgettable, life changing, love evolving experience. And no matter where we finish our race, I will always be glad we retied our laces!

FINAL COUNTDOWN

19th March 2021
EEEEK WE MADE IT!!! 37 weeks full term, writing this with Jovie still kicking away in my belly – Chris always told me Mannings are made of strong stuff!!!

I have woken up positive, thank goodness! Yesterday however had a completely different feel… panic set in and I went into overdrive about all the things I hadn't thought of and probably should of, I sent a mad amount of emails at 5am to different funeral directors, my midwife and people of support.

I remember this day well, I woke early as I just couldn't sleep from all the images running through my head of Jovie being left alone in a hospital morgue. Nightmares of her laying on a cold concrete slab, zipped up in a bag. I had even heard somewhere that baby's get incinerated in hospital or chucked in a grave with an old person. My mind was wild, I couldn't breathe, my heart was racing. Why hadn't I thought of this before? I believed that I was so organized and so prepared for all eventualities that it hit me so hard when I realised I had forgotten such an important detail. I was so angry with myself, I felt like I had failed Jovie.

I sent so many early morning, erratic, crazy emails, the recipients must have thought I had really lost it this time. But my impatience set in and as soon as the clock turned 9am I was on the phone to the funeral directors. They must have thought I was an absolute lunatic, planning my baby's death when she hadn't even been born yet! But they were so kind, they listened to my fears and spoke softly to me, they went through in depth about what happens when a baby passes away and they assured me that they did not get zipped in a bag or put on a concrete slab! Thank goodness, my heart warmed a little and I was able to breathe again! They informed me that I had choices *(you must know by now I like choices, and the need to be in control when it comes to Jovie)* and that she could stay with us for as long as we liked, either in hospital, in a hospice or at home. When the time came she could then be transported in a moses basket, which thankfully was far away from the thoughts I was having – my tiny new born baby on a metal trolley, rolling around in the back of a van!

Emails were sent back and forth to the hospital throughout the day, I needed them to know our wishes for our daughter and that under no circumstances was she going to a hospital morgue to be incinerated! I think they had already got the gist by now that I was having my baby, my way, but I just needed to make sure.

After I got my mind more settled of those thoughts no sooner did other thoughts kick in. I had spoken so much of her death but had I advocated enough for her life? What if she was born breathing? What if she was going to defy the odds? Did they know we wanted them to give her a fighting chance? Did they know that she deserved as much care as any other baby?

This is pretty much how that day went – a full on panic attack from start to finish, so I was glad when I woke up to week 37 feeling much calmer.

We tried to fill the next few days with positivity, embracing every second with our daughter still growing in my belly. We arranged a beautiful maternity photo shoot in the woods, done by a fellow photographer, photos I knew we would always treasure.

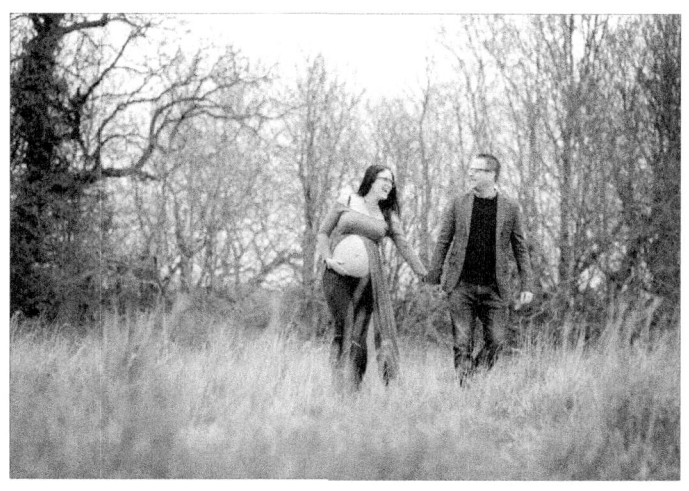

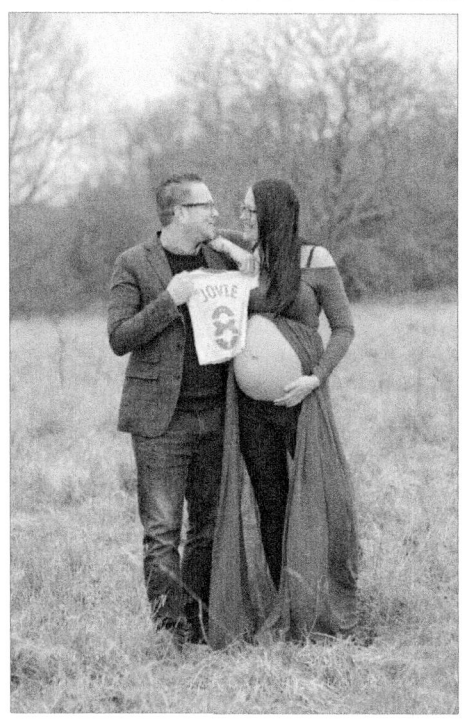

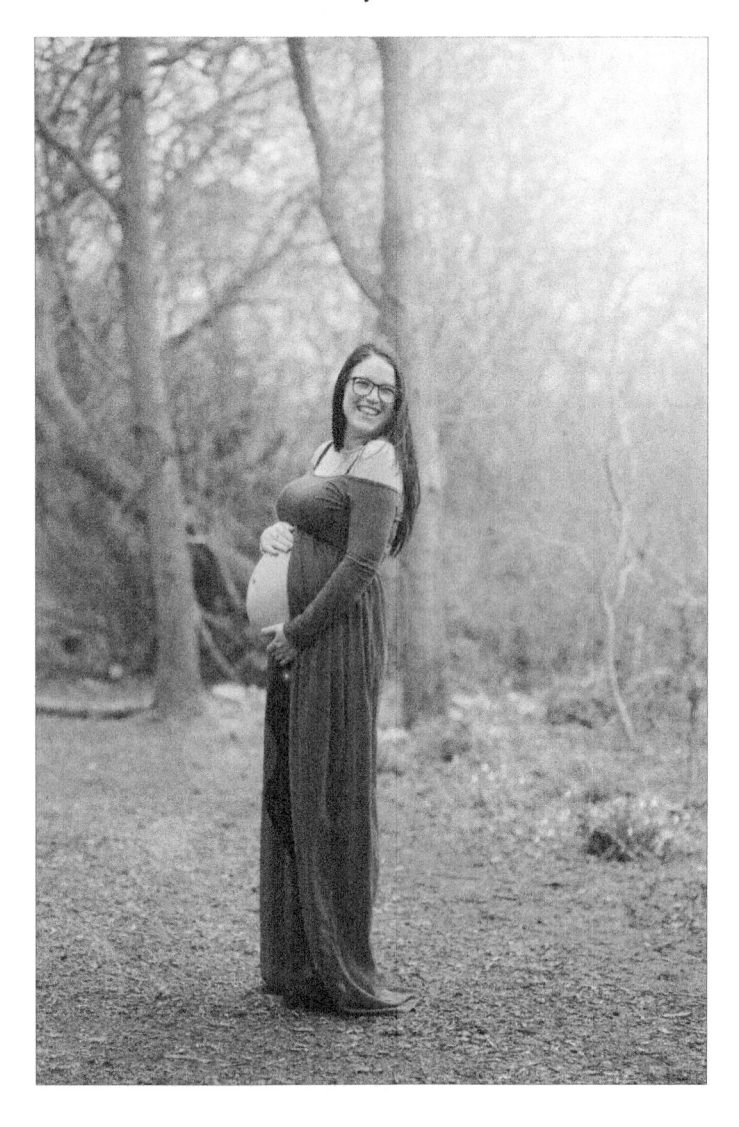

25th March 2021
Scan day again today! Now weighing approx 6lb 14oz, they are still happy with the performance of the cord and placenta and she is head down. We got to have a look around the bereavement suite, so is nice to be able to visualize those. Again no photos of her face as she had both of her fists up this time, she's definitely a fighter! Once again hospital have been amazing, we never feel rushed and nothing is ever too much hassle for them. Overall a positive appointment! I guess the rest is now down to Jovie x

26th March 2021
Day 266 of loving our little Jovie – aka 38 weeks! Still have to pinch myself we have made it this far… please don't be sad for us and the situation, no matter what happens we are having a baby in the next couple of weeks! Our daughter, created with love and who will know nothing but love and has made the meaning of love evolve beyond imaginable.

When I posted that last blog onto her Facebook page, I actually knew exactly when we were going to meet Jovie (unless she decided to come earlier of course!) However, even though we had chosen to make her journey public – and I should add here, it really was public now, word of the page had spread globally and people were rooting for her from across the globe – we felt we needed to keep this bit for ourselves. Knowing what might be to come, it was important for us to only have to share news in our own time without the pressure of people asking for updates, so we agreed only my parents and the children were to know.

It was decided that I would be induced, not an easy decision to make. It was totally against the plan for my natural birth, however, the hospital really wanted her born on a week day between 9am and 5pm, to give us more chance of the specialist medical team being on hand to care for her. The hospital had been so great at accommodating all of my wishes up until now, that I really felt I should listen to them on this one, and with all of the Easter bank holidays coming up around our due date it seemed the sensible thing to do. Not to mention the April Fools Day that was looming – whilst we had a good sense of humour , the thought of giving birth to a child with no life expectancy and one whom was expected to look *different* , on a day such as that, was something we wanted to avoid where possible. Our medical team were hopeful that with four previous births, the induction process would happen easily and it would progress naturally after that. I did put a few rules in place though! I was to remain mobile and I would not allow any unnecessary monitoring or examinations and everyone was to be on board with my hypnobirthing. Our hospital team prior to birth were pretty incredible, I don't know if they just figured out quite early on that I was a head strong woman who knew what she wanted so they didn't even bother to argue, or whether they were actually on board and trusted in my body as much as I did. I like to think it was the latter.

HAPPY BIRTHDAY

Tuesday 30th March, 2021, 38 weeks and four days pregnant – induction day! Jovie had come so far, from our first scan when we were told she had no face and told she would not survive pregnancy, being deemed "incompatible with life", being offered a termination, to now reaching full term – she had done it! Already defying all the odds, Jovie had made it to the end of the pregnancy and was ready to start her earth side story, however long or short that was going to be.

From the very first scan, we had always been open and honest with the children about Jovie. They were fully aware about all the uncertainties that surrounded the pregnancy, the chances of her passing whilst she was in my belly and the likelihood that she would not take a breath on the outside world. They knew she was going to look different and it was likely that when they eventually got to meet her she would probably already be in her forever sleep. So when the time came to leave for the hospital and say goodbye to the children, it was incredibly tough and emotional. We took last minute photos of them all with my pregnancy bump, kissed them goodbye and left them in the capable hands of my parents. All holding our breath that the next time we walked through our front door, by some miracle, we would have a baby in our arms.

The journey to the hospital was a weird one. We were calm and excited, but absolutely petrified of what was to come. To some extent we had lived in a little pregnancy bubble with Jovie safe and warm, growing nicely inside of me, I wanted to turn the car around and stay in our bubble forever.

We arrived at the hospital and parked the car like so many times before, only this time not knowing how long we would be leaving it there for. We made our way up to the ward, every possible thought was running through my head, but mainly anxiety about having to give birth in hospital, the last time I did that it was horrendous and I had grown to love the comfort of home births.

We were warmly greeted on the ward and showed to a side room where we had to wait a little while. They knew my wishes to have a water birth and I was keeping everything crossed the room with the pool in was free. You can imagine my delight when they come in and told us it was available. I hadn't even been induced by this point, but I think they were trying their upmost to make it the best possible experience for me, so allowed us to move straight into the pool room. Other than being at home, it really was the best I could have wished for. It was a nice big room with dimmable mood lighting, a sound system for soothing music and an en suite. It also had a bed, an armchair; unfortunately not the comfy sort but one of those that are typical for hospitals, which was also to be Chris' place to sleep, and a beautiful big bath; more like a Jacuzzi, with coloured lights and water jets. I set to work making it feel as homely as possible, with my chosen playlist on and my birth affirmations pinned up around the room.

At 1.30pm the induction process began, they opted for a mechanical induction with a balloon insertion. Basically in untechnical terms, they placed a balloon inside my cervix and slightly inflated it to put pressure onto the neck of the womb. The idea being that this should start contractions. Once the balloon was in the plan was to stay as mobile as possible and help things along as much as we could. I did some bouncing on the birthing ball and we went for a long walk around the hospital grounds. It was only March but it was a beautiful day, the sun was shining and there felt an air of positivity.

The day was passing us by and not a lot was happening in terms of my pending labour. I had a few mild contractions and by 9.30pm the balloon fell out on it's own. I think this was supposed to happen, it means my cervix had opened some more, but sadly not enough to start my labour. It was decided that they wouldn't do anything else to encourage it that evening and we would start again the next day, after all they ideally wanted her born in the day time.

I remember we didn't get much sleep, well Chris certainly didn't in his arm chair! But the morning of Wednesday 31st March arrived and we were greeted by our new midwife named Molly. She was a recently trained Midwife but filled me with absolute confidence, the way she showed full interest in my birth plan and my wishes for hypnobirthing was really entrusting. She didn't seem scared or worried for what she may be about to face, at least she didn't show this to us, instead she treated the day for what it was; the day we were about to meet our daughter. No matter what was going to happen later, together Molly, Chris and I were going to create the perfect birth.

I had requested minimal vaginal checks as they can have a detrimental effect to your mind set and make you feel you aren't progressing enough, and I didn't want to stay hooked up to a monitor for too long as staying active is key to a good birth. Molly broke my waters at 9am, I had to stay on a monitor for a short time to check Jovie's heartbeat was still regular but I was soon up and about again. By 10.30am I was having regular contractions.

My hypnobirthing practice taught how to feel "calm and relaxed" and to maintain this feeling there were certain rules in place. It had been agreed that the room would remain quiet, I would be allowed to go to my "happy place" with my head phones in, reading through my affirmations and moving around freely in the beautiful candle lit room. If anything needed to be discussed it would be done through Chris and I would not be disturbed. Chris and I had discussed at lengths how I wanted our birth experience to be and I had full trust in him that he would make all of the right decisions throughout. This was so important as it allowed my mind to be relaxed and my body to feel safe enough to allow my baby to move down the birth canal. In my mind I was a cow, birthing freely in a field.

Unfortunately, Doctor Alistair, who we had seen throughout our pregnancy and who had grown to know us very well was not on the ward that day. Had he been on the ward I know for certain the following incident would not have occurred. Despite it being in all my notes and the staff being fully briefed on our situation and birth plan, another doctor decided he knew best. He stormed into our room, completely breaking my zen and demanded that he needed to talk to me. He did not take any time to get to know us, ask how my labour was progressing (and it was doing pretty darn good!) or ask about our feelings. Instead he abruptly told me that if I wanted any chance of seeing my baby alive then I had to have a caesarean section. He went on to say if I didn't opt for a c-section right now then I would end up with an emergency one where I would have to be put to sleep, and therefore would miss any chance of seeing my baby! I was absolutely taken back that he felt he had the right to not only come into my room uninvited, ignore what Molly and Chris tried to tell him about discussing things with Chris first, and then go on to act like he knew what was best for me and my baby despite never having even met me before!

I could feel my eyes filling with tears, my heart started to race and every bit of safety that I had felt prior disappeared in a heartbeat. After a few seconds of panic our hypnobirth teaching kicked in, and Chris and I remembered what we had been taught about the right to choice and the right to question. We asked if he had anything related to my labour to back up what he was saying, which he didn't, and then we politely asked him to leave the room so we could discuss it with one another. He reluctantly left. Needless to say there was no discussion between Chris and I about the c-section. Chris and I both knew my labour was progressing nicely and Molly had not once expressed any concerns either. I explained to Molly that I did not want to see that doctor again, to which we never did! I have never been so grateful than I was in that moment for my hypnobirth teaching and for the trust Molly had in my body and her midwifery skills. For a newly qualified midwife to stand up to a doctor for the good of her patient, is just unforgettable. We will forever love you Molly.

It was now 1.10pm, thankfully I had managed to restore my zen and I allowed Molly to do a vaginal examination. In less than three hours from my first contraction I was already 7cm dilated. This just reinstated what I already knew about the power of a woman when mind and body can work together. I hope Molly delivered that bit of info to the doctor and shoved it up his arse!

Despite not being fully dilated, I knew I was getting close to delivering our baby. Until then I hadn't felt any pain and was embracing the labour. But the transition stage came, a stage I am sure a lot of birth mothers can relate to, when all rational thinking goes out the window and you scream for an epidural! I could literally feel Jovie clawing her way down my birth canal. Thankfully Chris was part of the hypnobirthing lessons too and he knew to expect this, this was where his role was really paramount. He had it drummed into him for months that no matter what I screamed, I did not want an epidural, instead he was to bring me back down to earth with calm words and positive affirmations. Thanks to Chris it only lasted a short while and I was back in the field, birthing freely like a cow!

I just want to say, I have nothing against c-sections, epidurals or pain relief, they are just not for me. My first birth I took all the pain relief available to me and it made me have the worst, longest, most drawn out birth ever, and I vowed I never wanted to go through that again. Having had both medicated and natural births, I just knew a natural birth was what I needed and if Jovie was going to have any chance of survival, she needed me to be as calm and relaxed as possible, and for me this is how that birth looked. What I do feel strongly about is that women know they have choices during birth, that they have the right to question doctors and that they should feel empowered enough to trust in their body and demand what they know is best for their body and their baby. I highly recommend the art of hypnobirthing, it can support any birth choices, including c-sections. The course I followed was *The Wise Hippo by Your Side for Bump, Birth and Baby* – if you are pregnant be sure to look it up. You really can have a pain free (almost, minus the small amount of clawing) birth!

As I knew it was getting close, at 1.18pm I got in the birthing pool. The water was warm and comforting and supported the weight of my bump. Before I knew it I was reaching down to feel Jovie's head enter into the world, at 1.48pm our beautiful baby daughter was born. I scooped up her little body with my own hands and placed her to my chest. Rapidly scanning her whole body with every sense I possessed, trying to take in every little piece of her, her smell, her feel, her looks, counting her fingers and toes, all in the matter of seconds. I glanced a look at Chris, his eyes filling with tears, he was the only one that truly understood the shear amount of emotion I was feeling in that moment; hope, gratitude and fear but mainly the overwhelming sense of love. A love like no other we had ever felt before, whatever we had already been through up until now and whatever we were about to face, this very second was worth every bit of it. She was perfect, we were complete and she was our daughter.

It had escaped me until that moment that a team of medical professionals were waiting outside the door ready for Jovie's impending entrance into the world. I suddenly felt their presence around the pool and saw them through teary eyes. The words left my mouth "Is she breathing? Do you need to take her?"

Their reply. "Yes she's breathing!"

She stayed placed on my chest and to my surprise they didn't take her, I was so elated as I never ever wanted to let her go. But why weren't they taking her? Were they just waiting for the inevitable so were giving us these precious moments with her? Did they not understand that if she came out breathing then our wish was for them to help her? Were they giving up on her already after she had fought so hard to be here? The answer to all of these was no, and we seemed to have full trust in their judgement. What they were doing was making their best empathic call based on our wishes, our birth plan and what was best for our daughter. They remained calm, were careful not to instil panic in us and carefully monitored the situation at the furthest distance they could, whilst allowing us this precious time as a family, after all she was breathing on her own.

Chris had been given strict instructions to film everything as I needed to know whatever time we had with Jovie was captured for us to relive again and again. (If you are interested in watching the birth video then you can find it on You Tube, just search *Our positive birth story – with Holoprosencephaly diagnosis*) I know he was torn between recording these precious moments as they unfolded but also being desperate to come round to my side of the pool to get a proper look at his daughter that he had been so eager to meet. He eventually was able to hand the camera to the nurse to come and meet his daughter properly. He knelt down behind me and cuddled into Jovie and I, with her still in my arms. That is a moment I will never forget. I am forever grateful for the pillar of strength Chris was throughout our pregnancy, the birth and still now. I could never have asked for a better partner to me or father to our daughter, than what Chris is. At risk of it sounding corny, he really was and is my rock, my best friend, my soul mate and the love of my life. I feel incredibly lucky that I get to call him mine.

We were now a good few minutes past birth, still in the pool and still in awe of our daughter breathing all by herself, we even got to hear her first little sound. As per our birth plan, we opted for delayed cord clamping as this serves all sorts of benefits to a newborn baby right up to the age of six months. Chris decided he did not want to cut the cord so the doctor did it instead and checked she was definitely a girl at the same time! It was then decided that they would take Jovie to the resuscitaire which was placed in the corner of the room, to check her over. I think everyone was in shock at how amazing she was doing, they had all expected the worst yet here she was showing them who was boss. I also think they were amazed at how beautiful she was, not just in terms of how she looked but the aura that came with her. I always knew she would be perfect to me, but it was very much expected for her to look different to a "normal" baby. I had made sure everyone in that room had been prepped for how different she may look as the last thing I wanted to see was shocked faces or hear mutters amongst those in the room. But I didn't see or hear anything of the sort. The room was full of love, kindness and amazement for this beautiful little miracle I had just brought into the world, and it was still so calm. You would imagine a room with at least eight to ten medical professionals in, two worried parents and a baby with a severe medical condition, to be loud and frantic with lots of rushing around where every second is crucial, but the reality was quite the opposite to this.

They were incredible, they had read my birth plan word for word, they understood my vision, whether they believed in it or not they seemed to trust what we had requested for our baby to be right. I like to hope their eyes were opened that day to textbook versus reality, and how their professional practice really can be adapted to take into account the wishes of the parents. But more importantly actually see how a calm environment with Mum being able to feel safe, is crucial to ensure a positive outcome for the birth and baby. Our gratitude goes out to both Helen and Florence who headed that team, for making the post birth experience everything we wished for, and for their continued care for Jovie.

The people in the room that day that got to witness a real life miracle and I'm pretty sure they finished their shifts as changed medical professionals. Jovie had pathed the way for better practice of complex births going forward. Our daughter was already fulfilling her purpose.

Assisting Jovie with a small amount of oxygen, they passed Jovie back to Chris and I for some snuggles. They had placed an adorable red knitted hat on her head for warmth. Immediately Mummy instinct kicked in and I wanted to be the one caring for Jovie, so I took over holding the little oxygen mask and gently placed it over her mouth and nose. Lots of photos were taken and we were just embracing every second of the three of us being together. My contractions then started again for the delivery of the placenta, so Chris had the perfect opportunity for his own skin to skin cuddles. I never realized I could love Chris any deeper than I already did until I saw him holding our daughter, and that just took it to a whole new level.

As much as I would have loved that moment to last forever, Jovie needed to be taken to the neonatal intensive care unit, for full assessment. Chris never left her side and stayed with her every step of the way.

<u>31st March 2021</u>
Today our beautiful baby girl Jovie, entered the world at 13.49pm weighing 7.12lb. We couldn't have asked for a more perfect birth, breathing on her own and continuing to defy all odds as she has done the whole pregnancy. Currently in NICU, taking each hour as it comes, but we feel the luckiest Mummy and Daddy alive right now to have already made so many memories with her. She is simply perfect and we are so in love.

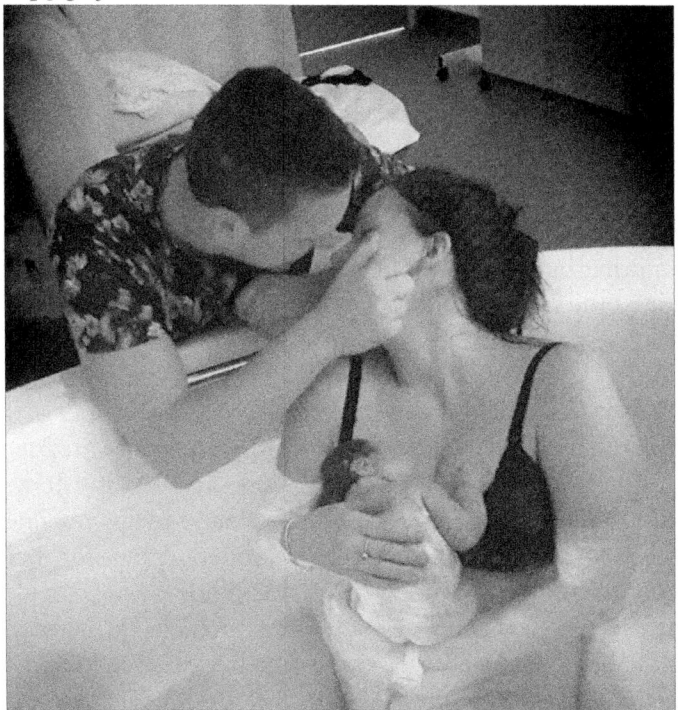

NICU

After what seemed like the longest fifteen minutes of my life, where I rushed to get cleaned up and my body back to some quick state of togetherness, I hurried to NICU to find Chris and Jovie.

The neonatal intensive care unit was adjacent to the delivery suite, through some double doors and across the corridor. On that first visit it didn't even cross my mind how much this place was going to become home over the upcoming days and weeks. At this point we still had no idea if Jovie was going to survive the next hour, let alone anything more.

I found Chris next to Jovie's bedside in room one, the high dependency unit. There were about six other incubators in the room, not all with babies in, and Jovie was in the first incubator on the right. Nothing can prepare you for the first time you see your baby in an incubator. Linked to various monitors, with so many wires, constant beeping either from her machine or another baby's, only able to look through perspex at this tiny little human you have been so desperate to hold for so long and unable to scoop them up into your arms like all your Mummy instincts want to do. Chris said she had been doing well, they had even taken her off oxygen already and replaced it with some pressured air through a little tube into her nose. I say nose, but Jovie didn't technically have a nose. She had a major midline cleft lip and palate, with only one opening for her mouth and nose, and no nostrils. I don't know if it's because I had prepared myself so much throughout pregnancy that she was going to look different or just the pure gratitude I had that she was even here and breathing, but I can honestly say I never ever looked at Jovie with shock or sadness, I never saw her deformities in a negative light, I only saw my beautiful and perfect little baby girl.

Jovie was born with the most gorgeous head of really dark brown hair, along with her eye shape she almost looked of Chinese origin. She was completely different to any of our other blonde children. But all that hair meant at just two hours old she had to have her first hair cut! Thankfully there was so much of it you couldn't notice too much, but they needed to remove some hair so they could fit tiny electrical pads to her head. She had these on until the following afternoon so they could measure any seizure activity her brain was having. The assessment showed that she was having both electrical and clinical seizures. Due to her diagnosis of Semi-Lobar Holoprosencephaly they said she would always have electrical seizures as her brain just wasn't wired up in a neurotypical way, however they started her on some medicines for the clinical seizures.

What was so heart warming about Jovie's first few hours in NICU was the buzz she had created around the hospital. She literally entered the world to her own fan club. We had done so much planning for Jovie's birth that everyone knew who she was before she was even born. All of the medical professionals that had met us along our pregnancy journey and even some who had just heard our story, were so eager to come and meet her. Maybe for some it was curiosity, but for most it was a genuine feeling of happiness and relief that our baby girl had made it, they were in awe of our real life miracle. The tears in their eyes couldn't lie.

When we arrived at the hospital about 36 hours earlier, I came loaded with my colostrum harvest! As I handed it over to the midwife for her to put in the freezer, I knew it was only wishful thinking that my baby was ever going to need it, but I tried to remain hopeful that all my efforts hadn't been in vain. Well, at 1am on 1st April, almost twelve hours after Jovie had been born, she received her first feed and it was all my mummy milk. Through her oral gastric tube Jovie received pure liquid gold, nature's best medicine, and I felt so proud I had been able to do that for her. I have breastfed all of my children, but never did I appreciate the value of it more than I did in that moment. Jovie tolerated her feed well, so two hourly feeds of 5ml of my colostrum continued throughout the night, with it soon being upped to 11ml. Though I came armed with a frozen stash of my milk, I knew it wouldn't last for long and I started expressing immediately. As a mummy in NICU you are pretty much stripped of all the normal mummy things you should be doing for your baby, so to be able to do this gave me a sense of purpose and I felt useful. It was hard graft, anyone that has exclusively expressed will know it is no mean feat to keep up with demand. Expressing every two hours throughout the night and day, I was exhausted, but with Jovie doing her part, the least I could do was mine.

With the high demand for the birthing pool on the delivery suite, we were asked to vacate our room. The staff were all keen for us to be able to stay at the hospital with Jovie as it was still thought that she was likely to pass away at any time, and there was no way we would be leaving her side. However, there were no parent rooms available on NICU and the only room left on the delivery suite was the bereavement suite. I knew what that room was, we had looked around it during a visit prior to the birth. It was a beautiful large room with a huge king size bed, a separate comfy seating area, it's own little kitchen and an en suite, a far cry away from any usual hospital room. But that's because it was a room made to feel as welcoming and homely as possible for the sole reason of spending quality time with your baby that has heartbreakingly passed away. This was the room we prayed we would never have to use. Whilst the staff knew it was far from ideal for our situation, there was no other option if we wanted to stay with our baby. I stood outside the door, tears filling my eyes, hands trembling, rooted to the spot. Whilst I was so grateful we weren't using it for the purpose of bereavement, I felt an overwhelming sense of emotion for all of those other poor parents that weren't as lucky as us. I knew our story could have been so different and I also knew it still could be.

After a bit of a wobble and a few deep breaths, I put my big girl pants on and we went in. We familiarized ourselves with the room and unpacked a few bits. Upon opening the wardrobe my heart broke all over again. There hung the most sweet and delicate little outfits, some so tiny that they would have even been too big for a doll. Then there, in the base of the wardrobe, intricately woven baskets of different sizes, inlayed with the softest cosiest bedding. Time felt like it stopped as I stood there staring into the wardrobe as I processed all of the emotions that had built up over the last couple of days and all of the thoughts of what we had to come. Chris eventually broke my trance, closed the wardrobe door, and we hurried off to be with Jovie again.

Our first full day on NICU was all a bit of a blur, so

many professionals wanted to speak to us and assess Jovie. We met the team from EACH, East Anglia's Children's Hospice, whilst they did explain their role to us, I'm not sure we took too much of it in. Still being the height of Covid-19 and hospital safety regulations being so strict, everyone was still wearing masks. As someone who is hard of hearing anyway, receiving an influx of information which just seemed foreign at times and then not being able to lip read, really made it quite difficult to process. We also met with Tracy, Jovie's assigned cleft specialist. She travelled from a different hospital a couple of hours away to assess Jovie's suck, swallow and gag reflex. With the deformation of Jovie's mouth, nose and airway, we could only hold our breath for some good news. Thankfully she passed all three with flying colours which meant it was safe to try and give Jovie a bottle. However, it wasn't a case of normal bottle feeding for Jovie. We had to learn a process called "teet nudging" and take things very slowly. By 3.30pm though, she had her first amount of mummy milk through a bottle, we were the proudest parents ever! Jovie would still continue to receive her milk via her oral gastric tube but the plan was to slowly combine the two. I even began to wonder if my dream of being able to breastfeed her may even become an option too. Either way, having got to give our daughter a bottle, change her bottom and even get her dressed meant we were winning!

1st April 2021
"…She is just a miracle and bossing everything they never thought she would do!...We have been so elated and floating on cloud 9 since the moment she arrived, we are so in love. But today has been full on at full speed, surviving on adrenaline and no sleep, but tonight I feel I am now crashing. We prepared ourselves so

much for the worst that now she is doing so amazing it feels scary and we haven't prepared for this feeling. It is such early days and we are so happy to take every memory she is giving us but we are trying not to be too complacent. Our mind keeps drifting to all the things we may actually get to do with her but we keep trying to rein it in as things can change very quickly in NICU. For now we are taking it hour by hour and keep cheering her along as does everyone else here.

Our baby girl Jovie, we couldn't ask any more of you, we love you so much and you are showing the world why us letting you tell your own story was the only and right choice.

As I have previously mentioned Jovie was born into a worldwide pandemic, despite some restrictions lifting, the hospital was still very much a controlled area. Chris was only allowed to be at the birth because of the severity of Jovie's prognosis and visitors were an absolute no no. It was always a big worry of ours that the children may never get to see their baby sister, but the staff at the hospital were determined to make it happen. It all became a bit of a secret undercover operation. It was a very sensitive subject for so many new parents on the delivery suite and in NICU, and rightly so. Women were being forced to go through labour without their partner and dads were missing out on seeing their child enter the world. All the babies in NICU were there because they required extra support, so why should any allowances be made for us? The truth is, most of those babies were going to be going home to have a lifetime with their families, ours was not. Jovie was still in very much a critical condition and needed constant monitoring, so it wasn't just a case of sneaking her into another room, she would need monitors and a nurse with her at all times. Thankfully we were still staying in the bereavement suite at the time which happened to be the last room at the end of the corridor on the delivery suite, conveniently placed next to an exit door out into the main area of the hospital. This meant it would be easier to sneak the children in without anyone seeing them. It really did feel very naughty and of course we didn't want to put anyone in the hospital at risk of catching Covid-19, but the staff weighed up the pros and cons, risk assessed the whole situation and were happy for it still to go ahead.

On 2nd April, with much care and precaution, a whole load of face masks and PPE, very quiet tiptoes and no talking until fully inside the room, a mobile monitor for Jovie and a very understanding Nurse - Jovie met her brothers and sisters! It was a moment we or them will never forget. They fell in love with her immediately and I fell deeper in love with this beautiful family we had created. Jovie was the glue that stuck our two blended families together. As the children couldn't drive themselves to the hospital and they couldn't all fit in one car, it was the perfect excuse for both my parents and best friend to come too. As much as we wish that moment could have lasted forever we were also very aware of how lucky we were that it could even happen at all, so a quick cuddle for each of them with Jovie and a quick cuddle with each of them for us and they were ushered out of there as secretly as they came in. Seeing the children really was the emotional charge we needed, as being apart from them was an additional strain.

Since the moment Jovie had been born we had not left her side, other than the odd hour or two when our bodies would finally give in for some sleep. On 3rd April she had some medicine which made her very sleepy, it was so they could assess her a bit more without it causing any distress. The nurse convinced us to use this opportunity to go and get some fresh air whilst Jovie was sleeping, reluctantly we did. Knowing that things could change any second, and knowing our seconds with her were limited, we didn't want to miss a single one but the fresh air on our faces really did feel good! Being a chocoholic, I was seriously feeling the withdrawal symptoms of a few days without any, so we decided to take a quick drive to the local Tesco Express. It was literally a two minute drive away so we knew we could be there and back in a flash. We popped in Tesco, loaded up with chocolate and got back in the car. Being how anxious we were leaving Jovie I have absolutely no idea why or how both of us managed to leave our phones in the car. When we looked at them before driving off we saw we both had missed calls from NICU, our hearts left our body and full panic mode set in. Chris tried to call them back as I sped the two minute drive back to the hospital, whilst it felt the longest drive of my life I am sure I managed it in thirty seconds. The ward hadn't answered our call back so we literally stopped the car in the first place we could find, jumped out and ran up to the ward. Frantically ringing the door bell and screaming down the intercom to let us in, we burst through the doors and went straight to Jovie's incubator, where it was unexpectedly calm. The nurse was at her bedside as we blurted out "What's wrong with her, we missed your call, what's happening to her?" Her reply, "She was rooting for you, so I called you as thought you would want to put her to the breast". What was I hearing? I nearly just killed us and everyone in our path driving like a mad woman to get back, all because Jovie was rooting? The poor nurse, she was so apologetic, I think she could see from our faces the sheer fright she had put in us. Once I had managed to breathe again and felt my body reminding me that I had only given birth three days prior and running that marathon really wasn't a bright idea, I took in exactly what was happening here. This nurse that had just scared me half to death, over the last few days must have really listened and understood the yearning I had to breastfeed my daughter. So as soon as she saw Jovie giving the cues, knowing how much it meant to me and that I wouldn't have wanted to miss the opportunity for the world, decided to ring me. It was so heart warming that she understood the importance of me putting Jovie to the breast, even though she knew Jovie was getting her milk through a tube anyway. I could not show that nurse my gratitude enough, and my only hope is that one day she gets to read this so she knows how that moment will stay etched in my heart forever.

Due to Jovie's severe midline cleft she was unable to form enough suction around my nipple to actually feed from me, but from that moment on putting her to the breast for her comfort was something we did often. As time went on we experimented with a supplemental nursing system, so she could also tube feed from the breast – but that's a good Google for you if you are interested!

Like every day in NICU, great highs are followed by great lows. We were sadly told that we were no longer able to stay in the bereavement suite as it was required by another family and there were still no rooms on NICU for us. We were absolutely devastated, but how selfish we were for feeling sad that we no longer had a bed, when the reality was it meant some other poor parents had lost their baby. NICU had 24 hour access to parents, so our plan was to just sleep by her bedside, though I'm not sure how maintainable that would have been when it didn't even have an armchair. Thankfully, someone was looking over us, as before the day was through a room became available in NICU, we were able to stay after all.

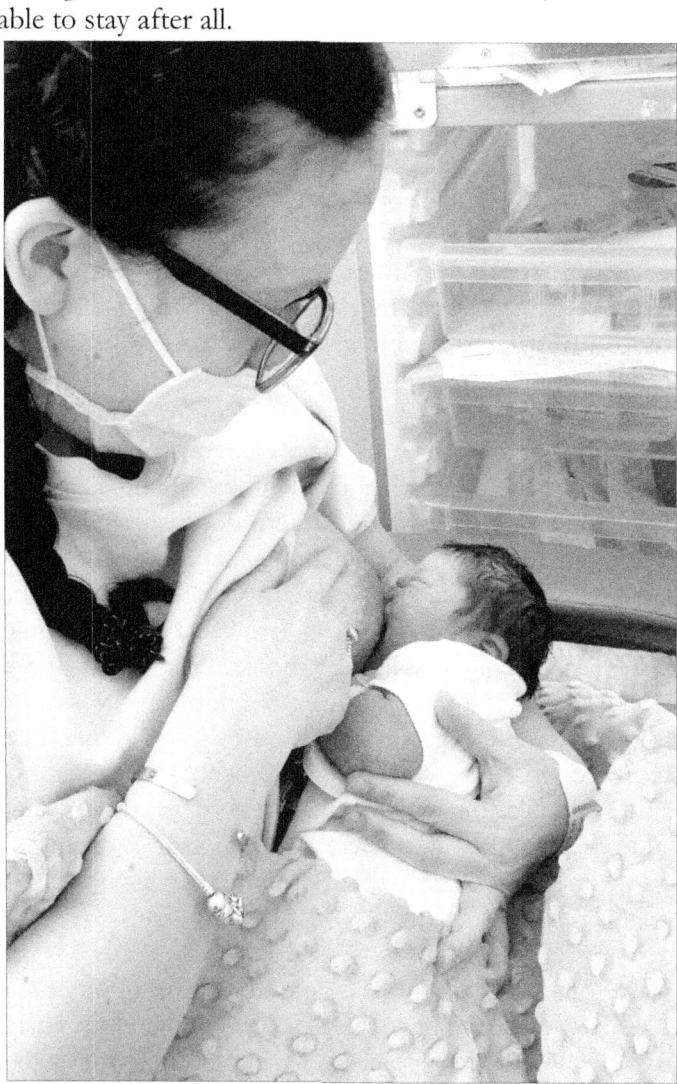

NICU is a whole little world of its own, it becomes your home and the staff become your family. It is made up of a front desk, room one, two and three, from high dependency through to getting ready to go home, an emergency medical room, parent bedrooms, a milk kitchen, a freezer room to store expressed milk and a parent kitchen and lounge.

Room one, high dependency, was very quiet other than the constant beeping of monitors. The babies in there were very poorly so it had a solemn air around it and no one tended to speak to each other. When the doctors needed to speak to parents about their baby, often bad news, a screen would be pulled around them to give a bit of privacy and ear buds would be handed out to the other parents. One thing that has always stuck with me was a tiny baby, the same side of the room as Jovie with an empty bay between us. The Dad was sitting beside the incubator for a considerable about of time reading the baby a story. I hadn't seen him do this before and I could just tell it was with such a heavy heart. The Mum joined him a little later, the doctor came and pulled the screen across, but even through my ear buds I could hear heartbreaking sobbing. We left the room for a while as we went with Jovie to another part of the hospital where she needed some tests. When we returned their bay was clear, the incubator was empty and it was like they were never there. A few hours later a new baby filled it's place. It didn't take a genius to work out the ending to that story and it hit us with a massive dose of reality.

Jovie only ever spent the odd day in room two, it seemed to be a more sociable room, the babies seemed to have found their voice and parents would chat and get to know each other. I've heard that many great friendships are formed in NICU but I only really got to exchange the odd conversation in the milk kitchen whilst waiting for Jovie's milk to warm. But I can't complain, the reason we weren't in room two much was because on 4th April, only four days after being born Jovie got promoted! She bypassed room two and three and moved straight into our bedroom.

4th April 2021
…Little Miss Jovie has only gone and graduated from Room 1 (high dependency / intensive care) into OUR ROOM! That's right, apart from her meds, her entire day to day care (including hourly feeds) is with us now…if she keeps this up we will be home before we know it!!! Obviously the doctors and nurses are still checking in and are there for serious seizures etc. but this is a massive step forward. Eeeeeek, a week ago we were counting down what we thought were our last days with her and here we are now celebrating her first Easter all together as our little family.

5th April 2021
…The word "home" has been mentioned, it's hard to allow ourselves to believe that we might actually get to take our daughter home one day, it's still quite a way off but there are goals to now work towards to get us on the right path. We may be tired, but we are the happiest and proudest parents alive.
…Jovie saw her first snow fall (from the hospital window) at 5 days old and in April – how very random!

6th April 2021
…I feel so totally blessed to have had our baby girl for 6 whole days and the luckiest person on earth to be sharing all these moments with the most incredible Daddy and boyfriend. Chris has been my rock through the whole pregnancy and is looking after us both perfectly. My heart is just overflowing with love for him, Jovie

and all of our children who we are missing so much. The day we are back together as a family will be one to remember.

7th April 2021
Jovie is 1 whole week old today! Cannot believe we get to say that, eeeek! She celebrated with her first bath and putting on her first dress… We are the proudest and happiest parents, she is just so scrummy and we find ourselves just sitting looking at her, praising each other on what a gorgeous baby we have made!

8th April 2021
Today Jovie is wearing tights for the first time as the monitor that attaches to her foot has gone! Mummy and Daddy just need to be brave now and trust in themselves to monitor her seizures by looking / listening to her and not by the machine, It may go back on tonight depending on how brave we feel! Once it's gone completely that will be another tick on the discharge list! Go Jovie!...

Today has been the hardest day so far since we've been in here. After feeling so elated for so long, the adrenaline that was keeping me going has now been replaced with tiredness and overwhelming emotion. What we have been through and what Jovie has to come has really hit home today. It hasn't helped that she has had one test after another today… inconclusive hearing test so have a further referral, blood tests and an EEG where she had nearly 30 electro pads stuck to her head for nearly 2 hours, having to watch her seizure and not be able to pick her up. On top of that she has vomited twice really bad today, throwing out her feeding tube both times, meaning more stress on having her having it put back in. She's not been left alone long enough to warm up meaning more seizures than normal. It's the worst feeling watching our baby girl have to undergo all this… on a positive note we did grab half an hour to leave these 4 walls and take her on a stroll around the hospital, was nice to see something different, even if it was just corridors, and put her in a pram for the first time. She is now snuggled up on my chest having skin to skin, much more chilled out. Hoping tomorrow isn't so stressful!

I had been keeping Jovie's Facebook page updated for family, friends and for everyone else across the globe who had been invested in her, to see how she was progressing. I always wanted her page to be a true representation of her journey, the highs, the lows and all the bits in between. I had reached 9th April 2021 without showing her face to the world, for many reasons really. I had made our journey and my emotions so public that I just wanted to keep a bit of her to myself. I knew she was beyond beautiful but she did look *different*, so maybe a little bit of me was scared of what people might say, the internet can be a cruel place. But on this day, I asked a doctor, "Do you see many babies with Jovie's condition?" and he replied "No. Well quite a few diagnosed in utero but most are terminated and not given the chance like Jovie." I knew in that moment that the world needed to see Jovie to fully appreciate why it was so right to give her a chance at life. She wasn't just a statistic, another baby, a deformity… she was our daughter and she was as perfect, beautiful and worthy of life as any other baby. At what stage are these text books going to be rewritten and the statistics updated? Surely if a baby isn't given a chance at life then these statistics that they spout at you during their termination speech are just plucked out of thin air? This "incompatible with life" saying is being used daily around the world and it scare mongers parents into aborting their baby, when the reality of it is when you look in the real world, there are babies, children and even adults, living, loving and thriving everyday with this so called "incompatible with life" prognosis. And the ones that don't make it to full term, or through birth or past a week old, what they give to their parents and what they can teach the world in their short time is invaluable. Here Jovie was at only 9 days old, yet she had taught me more about love, life, empathy and gratitude than I had ever learnt in my past 36 years. The world needs to sit up and realise that there are more ways to measure a life than these idealistic perceptions that people seem to hold onto, as the real meaning of life is deeper than any of those.

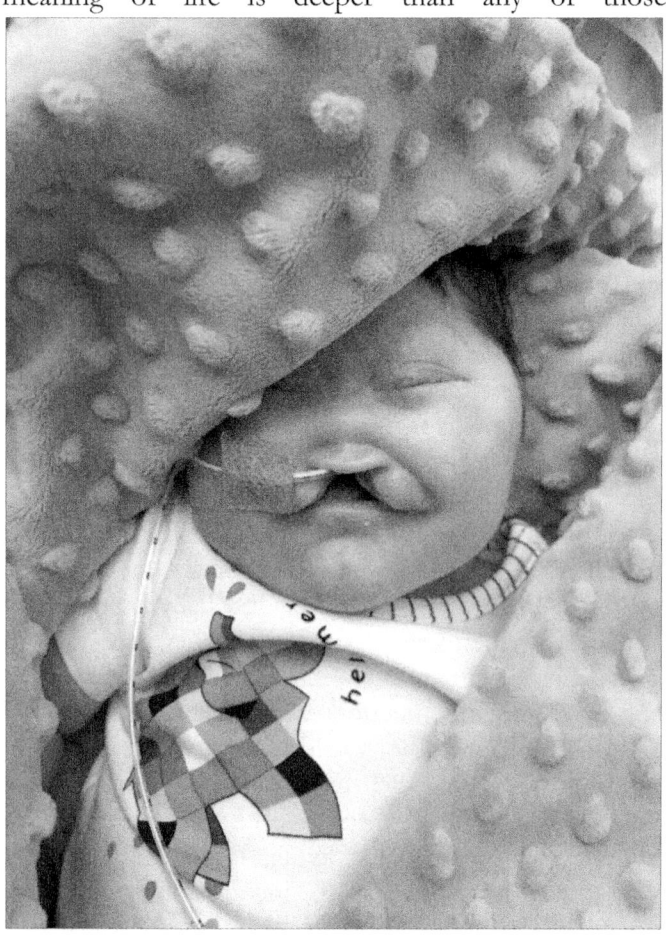

Life in NICU was starting to take it's toll. We would work our way through the "getting home" checklist;
- ✓ Car Seat Challenge
- ✓ No monitor
- ✓ Administering meds ourselves
- ✓ Placing the feeding tube ourselves

even be given a going home date as Jovie was doing so well, only to have it all ripped away. On 13th April, the night before our planned discharge date, Jovie took a turn for the worst, it was terrifying. One minute she was fine chilling with us in our room, the next she started making some scary gasping noises and completely zoned out. I knew something wasn't right and immediately called the doctor in. Jovie was rushed off into intensive care, it was all so manic and so frightening, so many people running around trying to save her, the whole time us not really knowing what was going on. The doctor asked us how much we wanted them to intervene to save her. Was this really happening? Was it the time we knew was going to come but hoped never would? Five minutes earlier she was absolutely fine, we were going home tomorrow, and now what, she was dying in front of our eyes? Of course we wanted them to save her, we weren't ready to say goodbye but at the same time we had always promised her and each other we wouldn't push her too far. Standing back helplessly watching doctors play God with our child's life, whilst we could do nothing but hope they believed in her as much as we did.

Thankfully, by some kind of miracle, Jovie pulled through without needing too much intervention. Only days before did we have to complete a Respect form about what sort of medical intervention we would want in an emergency. It was almost as if it was written for this to happen. The Respect form is something that has been changed and updated throughout Jovie's life, the more doctors and us have got to understand her capabilities and what fair boundaries are for Jovie. But it is always the hardest conversation to have and never gets any easier.

Jovie stayed in intensive care for a couple of days, it felt like the last two weeks hadn't even happened and we were back to square one. We were surrounded by beeping machines and watching screens be pulled across all over again and our bedroom felt so lonely without our little room mate.

Whilst Jovie was in intensive care part of her chromosome tests came back. She had been tested to see if it was genetics that had caused her brain condition, Holoprosencephaly. Throughout pregnancy they feared that she either had Trisomy 13 (Patau's Syndrome) or Trisomy 18 (Edward's Syndrome). As her brain condition was so severe they already deemed it fatal, however one of these syndromes could have caused other complications. Her tests came back negative for both, as well as for Down Syndrome, which we already knew about.

A week or so later we received the results of the other part of the tests. They were explained to us by another doctor that clearly didn't know Jovie well, I'm not sure from his comment whether he had even read her notes. He concluded that Jovie had 7q36.1q36.3 deletion. When asked what this meant for Jovie he replied "I'm really sorry but she won't be able to have children when she is older". Excuse me? Two weeks ago we were told she wouldn't even make it home and here you are telling us our baby girl won't have children? This was the frustrating part of NICU, doctors were on a three day rota. You would just get to know a doctor and they would get to know Jovie only for them to do a rota change. One would tell us they want to get you home tomorrow, the next would say home is months away. One would say she may not make it through the day, the next would say she can't have children. To put it bluntly, it was an absolute head fuck! Thankfully we did have one constant, we called her our NICU Mum, Sarah. She was our absolute angel; we would have never got through NICU life without her. She was there to wipe our tears, listen to our rants and keep everyone doing what they should be doing. Sarah has always kept an ear out for Jovie and often visits us when we are back in the hospital.

16th April 2021
I really do try and stay positive but it just feels so hard sometimes when home was in touching distance. I am so grateful for all this time we have had with Jovie that I didn't think we would get but being Mummy to her for 2 weeks and properly caring for her on our own, I just miss her not being with us so much. I just want her back with us and I want to take her home. When she got really poorly the other night it reminded us that we don't have her forever so I just want to spend it as a family. I just feel like I've hit a brick wall today.

Chris - "After this morning's little wobble Jovie had plans to move back into our room, no monitor needed and there is also the word home mentioned again. Me and Debz got super excited and had to take a trip out to buy the pram, exciting times we are just so happy to have her back in our room, extra cuddles and kisses"

17th April 2021
It actually feels pointless updating this page at the moment as everything seems to change so quickly. Yesterday we were out buying a pram excited that Jovie was coming home in a couple of days, today, home feels like weeks away. Life in NICU is so hard. I've never known something evoke so many different emotions over such a short space of time. I am tired, teary and missing my babies at home so much. Feeling torn between wanting the best care for Jovie but also wanting to spend the limited time she has at home as a family.

With the hopes of home being ripped away from us once again, the hospital granted us a very exceptional four hours leave, with Jovie! With our return journey being over two hours, it really was a flying visit, but it was so needed. We kept it a surprise, so when we walked through the door to my parents house where the children were staying, we were greeted with their biggest smiles and even some happy tears. Everyone was so excited to see Jovie, because the truth is, they never knew if they were ever going to get to see her again.

Before I had any children I had a dog called Dolly. She was a black and white Jack Russell crossed with a Lhasa Apso, she really was my world, my first baby and had been by my side through the whole of my adult life. She saw me through a marriage and the birth and lives of my three children. Dolly was still with us, though she was very old and starting to feel very sorry for herself. One of my biggest wishes through my pregnancy with Jovie, was that Jovie and Dolly would get to meet. I held out hope that Dolly would stay with us long enough to meet Jovie should a miracle happen. Well that miracle happened, because on the 18th April 2021, on our brief visit home, they met. Little did I know they were actually going to have many months of being the best of friends. Jovie even has "Dolly" as her middle name.

After visiting my parents' home we managed to squeeze in a visit to our house. Carrying Jovie through our front door was something we never thought we would get to do, but here we were doing it, another amazing milestone. Chris' children were there waiting for us, along with Jovie's other Nanny and Grandad. Jovie also met her big brother Keane for the first time (it was decided that because he was younger that he wouldn't come to the hospital when the others did). Jovie even got to open the Christmas present we had bought her when I was pregnant. The fun was short lived as it was soon time to go back to the hospital, we had promised them we wouldn't miss our four hour curfew!

Our further days in hospital were spent getting Jovie's medications right. It had become apparent that Jovie had Diabetes Insipidus, this is quite common in children with Jovie's condition. It was a tricky one to manage and we came to learn just how much impact sodium levels can have on the body. Jovie also continued to have seizures so the doctors were trying the best cocktail of medicines to manage these. We got Jovie's second hearing test back, it was good news, she did have some hearing. She couldn't hear quiet sounds and she had glue hear which muffled the noise for her, but that was something she would grow out of in years to come.

The up and down of NICU life continued, generally day to day with Jovie was just like having any neurotypical baby. She ate, she slept, she cried, she pooped and she loved her skin to skin cuddles with Mummy and Daddy. On 28th April however, she did give us another scare and ended up back in intensive care. She had began making rasping sounds and then went floppy whilst she had a prolonged seizure which lasted about two hours. After that she was fine again but had to stay in intensive care for 24 hours for them to monitor her – once again we were missing our room mate.

1st May 2023
Dear Jovie,
Thank you for proving to the world that you deserved to tell your own story, thank you for showing them your strength and your beauty but most of all thank you for allowing us to be your Mummy and Daddy and giving us so many memories with you already, we are the proudest parents on earth to have you as our daughter.

Happy one month old baby girl, this is what miracles are made of.

We love you x

The day had finally arrived, 7th May 2021, 38 days after we entered the hospital feeling anxious and ready to birth our baby, it was time to leave the place that had become home, the place that felt safe, the only place we had known with our daughter. Now it was time to go, armed with bags and boxes of medical supplies, feeding tubes, and medicines, it didn't feel like such a good idea after all. The reality of taking our severely medically complex baby home, who was still having many seizures, suddenly became petrifying. After saying our goodbyes to the staff that had become like family, we walked out of the Neonatal Intensive Care Unit doors with complete apprehension but with the biggest feeling of joy and gratitude that we had been blessed with this miracle. Driving home was the scariest drive of my life, it felt like I had never driven before, I was so aware of how precious the cargo was that I was carrying.

Our daughter did it, Jovie made it home.

HOME LIFE

We were home and had completed our family with our own little miracle, the thought of making it to this moment is what kept us going over the past five weeks in hospital and we finally made it. Normal life resumed almost immediately with Chris going back to work and myself having school runs to do. The children had some very proud moments pushing Jovie to school in her pushchair. Roux was particularly excited to be able to show her off in the playground and to his teacher, he certainly took well to the protective big brother role. This made me so happy that despite her looking different, she still had the proudest big brothers and sisters; they didn't even seem to question what others would think of her.

It was heartbreaking for Chris to leave Jovie and go to work, knowing that our time with her was still limited he really didn't want to miss any of it. It was also hard for me to let him go, the thought of being solely responsible for this fragile little life, managing feeds, medicines and seizures all on my own was extremely overwhelming. But it was our life now and we needed to embrace it, after all she continued to defy all odds, maybe just maybe she was going to be here to stay. Life just had to become a whole new normal.

Our new normal consisted of lots of appointments back at the hospital, especially in the early days as they were trying to explore all of Jovie's medical abnormalities, including spinal checks, EEGs, bloods, dieticians etc. Part of me liked going back to the hospital though, it felt safe there and as much as we were desperate to leave NICU I kind of missed it. NICU kept us embraced in its own little bubble, where all we had to worry about was Jovie, and Chris and I had all the time in the world for each other, in a weird way it was kind of bliss. Being thrown back into the chaos of everyday life suddenly made me realize how much I craved that bubble again.

Still determined to make every second count, we filled all of our family time together making memories. Things that we used to take for granted now became so special. A simple walk in the woods was now a carnival for my senses, the smells of being outside and the noise of the trees blowing in the wind, the children laughing together, it was all more acute than ever. The task of carrying Jovie in her sling as we walked amongst nature warmed my heart more than words can ever describe.

Life was certainly never dull with Jovie around, and she continued to have up and down days. The up days kept us grateful and the down days kept us from becoming complacent. Living on constant high alert became emotionally exhausting.

Her Story To Tell

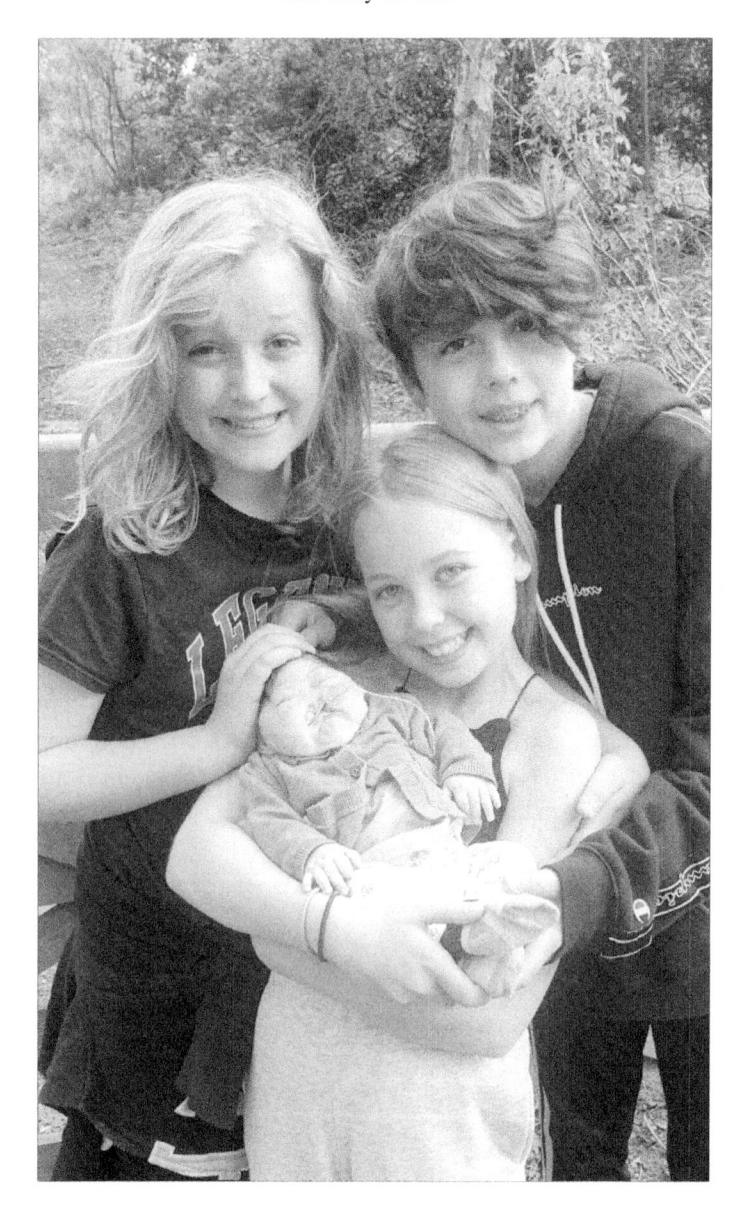

<u>23rd May 2021</u>
Too scared to close my eyes, I would rather watch you sleep,
As I hear you breathing faster, again I start to weep.
No one knows you like I do, they think now you're here you're ok,
But I've seen you getting paler, I know you've struggled today.
I put you on my chest, your favourite place to be,
It brings me comfort to feel you so very close to me.
I thought it would get easier now that pregnancy you made it through,
But every day the fear gets deeper, the fear of losing you.
You are the strongest little human and I know you're trying your best,
I just know the time will come when you need to rest.
Just remember my sweet Jovie how much Mummy loves you,
And no matter what you need I will always help you through.

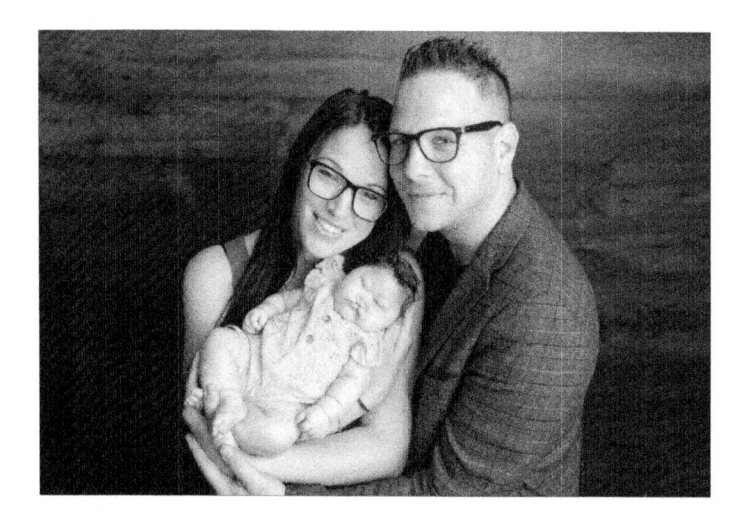

On 26th May, I had our first scary experience with Jovie since being home. I was on our usual school run with the children all loaded into the car and Jovie next to me in her car seat. That morning in particular we happened to be taking another little boy to school as well. I just pulled up at his house when Jovie was violently sick and her face turned completely purple. I quickly got her out of her car seat to stop her choking, her purple face then turned to white and she went all limp in my arms as she stopped breathing. Thankfully the Mum of the boy we were picking up took all of the children into her house so they didn't have to witness what was going on. After the longest four minutes of my life, which consisted of intense rubbing, back patting and gentle breathing into Jovie's mouth, she finally started to make a little noise and breath on her own again. After a couple more minutes she was back to normal and had her usual pink little cheeks back. I remained strangely calm, got the children back in the car and took them to school. As soon as I was back on my own with Jovie, the enormity of what just happened hit me. I began sobbing uncontrollably and I couldn't stop. The scary reality of keeping my baby alive, of keeping her from death, was my life now.

Thankfully, Jovie and I were making our way to the local hospital straight after the school run anyway as we had an appointment to get her blood gases done. There she was checked over, her SATS were normal and she kept a feed down fine, so we were allowed back home again. Unfortunately though it seemed that reflux which had possibly caused this, was becoming a problem and we started on a run of trial and errors to figure out what was causing it.

28th May 2021
…Jovie has had a really scary few episodes these last couple of days where she has stopped breathing for a considerable amount of time. So today we made sure "life" just waited and we took Jovie to feed the ducks, see the squirrels, go on the swings and put her feet in the sand. We did it with a smile on our faces as our daughter is still here with us, but tears in our eyes as we knew why we were so keen to make these memories today.

As part of one of my job roles as a Nursery Practitioner I have partaken in many paediatric first aid courses, and upon preparing to leave NICU they make sure they teach you how to perform CPR on a baby. When learning these new skills you always hope you will never have to use them, even with a severely medically complex daughter I didn't think I would ever actually have to do it. That was until the 31st May 2021, when for the fourth time in a week, Jovie stopped breathing again. Chris and I were both at home with her, despite me explaining her previous similar episodes to him, this was the first time he had witnessed it for himself, and this time it was worse than ever. It was hands down the single most scariest thing I have ever had to deal with up until that point in my life. No words can describe how helpless you feel as a mother, seeing your baby turn lifeless and floppy. I did all the usual things I had done before to get her breathing again but nothing was working. Minutes were passing, Chris and I looked at each other, knowing this time was different and almost to say who was going to do it. Chris flung his arms across the coffee table, clearing it of its clutter, as I placed Jovie down on the hard surface, "just do it" he exclaimed. As Chris called for an ambulance, I started pressing my two fingers down into Jovie's chest counting as I did so. This followed with placing my lips around her mouth and nose to form a seal, and blowing air into her tiny little lungs. Once again, although I was petrified I was losing my little girl in front of my eyes, a weird sense of calm and control took over me. If you had asked me before this moment who would be the calmest one to perform CPR out of Chris and I, I would have definitely said Chris every time, but my mummy instincts seemed to kick in and I just did what I needed to do.

I don't know how long this went on for, the world seemed to stop, but just as she started breathing again the ambulance people burst through the door. They checked her over and once more Jovie was back to her usual self, she seemed to have the best bounce back ability ever. The ambulance people said to us, had they not seen me doing CPR when they walked in they wouldn't have believed Jovie had just had a cardiac arrest. Cardiac arrest? Those words suddenly seemed massive and the reality of what just happened started to dawn on me.

Due to that big *word* that just happened, Jovie had to be taken by ambulance to the hospital. As I walked out of the house with Jovie in my arms I was shocked by the sight of what had unravelled outside. Our narrow road, lined with terrace houses from top to bottom, that even a normal sized car had to squeeze through, had been overtaken by three police cars and two abandoned ambulances that couldn't quite make it as far as our house. Apparently it's normal protocol for police to attend when a child has a cardiac arrest. It certainly gave the curtain twitchers of our road something to gossip about!

Unfortunately the ambulance people would only take us to the local hospital (the one that at our 12 week scan told us she had no face) and not our normal hospital of choice that really knew Jovie. Despite the hype of Covid-19 now being out of the media, hospitals were still very strict on their regulations and only one of us were allowed in the hospital with her, this never got any easier for either of us, whether we were the one with her or the one left behind. On arriving at the children's ward we were put in a side room on our own rather than the communal bay. Whilst I was grateful for the privacy, being met with the sudden loneliness made the past hour's events hit me like a tonne of bricks. I sat in floods of tears next to Jovie in the hospital cot, coming to the realization that I had just performed CPR on my own baby and that we had come so close to losing her. I wished so hard that a nurse, a cleaner, just someone, would come in and put their arms around me and just acknowledge this huge trauma I had just been through, or even just offer me a cup of tea. I cried, I waited, but no one came, not even to check on Jovie. Admittedly she was stable on arrival but she also had just had a cardiac arrest as they told me, along with her history that week of stopping breathing. This pretty much set the tone for this stay and all subsequent stays at this hospital. It only heightened my anxiety surrounding the care they were willing to provide Jovie and their unwillingness to get to know her. They had written her off from the start without even asking me her name.

One of the most vivid memories I have of this hospital came from this stay. After hours of being left alone, Jovie's named consultant for this hospital finally came in to see her. He was the consultant that had sat in the zoom calls during our stay in NICU, when all of the medical professionals that were to be involved in Jovie's care came together to discuss her. When he came in I was naively expecting "Hello, I'm Doctor … from the zoom meetings, nice to finally meet you, this must be Jovie" etc etc. I couldn't have been more wrong. Instead he walked in the room, did not introduce himself, glanced in the cot at Jovie and said "I'm happy for her to be discharged". No hello, no introduction, no assessment, just happy to discharge a baby who had only hours before had a cardiac arrest and whose Mother had gone through the biggest trauma of her life, yet he was happy for her to be discharged!!! I am damn sure had Jovie been a neurotypical baby with a full life expectancy, he would not have been so keen to discharge her so quickly.

As much as I did not want to be at that hospital with people who weren't willing to see what an amazing and worthy baby Jovie was, I was also fully aware that something was going on to cause these sudden episodes of Jovie stopping breathing, and I was not willing to take her home until I had got to the bottom of it. Had Jovie's named Consultant from the nice hospital (whom I am yet to give enough praise in this book) not been on annual leave, I would have walked out with her there and then and took her straight to him. But instead I had to stay and fight this fight for our baby girl.

Chris and I had discussed previously what could be causing these sudden respiratory episodes. We had put it down to the increase in one of her medicines, Clobazam. It is known to effect respiratory and there is a fine balance in getting it right. Her dose was increased just before they started happening, so it seemed obvious. I shared my concern with the nurses and doctors but no one seemed to take me seriously. They were not willing to decrease a medicine another doctor had prescribed, despite it nearly causing my daughter's death. But with Jovie's doctor on annual leave surely someone had to make a decision? The truth is, her named consultant at that hospital became disinterested in Jovie from the minute we expressed during the NICU zoom meeting, that we were keeping the majority of her care at the other hospital. He allowed his ego to interfere with getting to know Jovie, and denied Jovie her basic human rights of a fair shot at life.

With no one listening to me, after a couple of days of being in there I decided to take Jovie home. At least there we were the ones in control of Jovie's medicines and despite him being on annual leave Jovie's consultant from the other hospital called me and let me know of our choices in terms of her medicines. He supported us in our decision to reduce her dose of Clobazam and as expected the respiratory episodes subsided! I honestly believe if we had stayed in the hospital and left her on the higher dose, she wouldn't still be here.

We were quickly learning that we had to speak up and often question decisions if we thought they were wrong, if we wouldn't advocate for Jovie then who would? It's super hard, telling a doctor you think they are wrong, after all they have trained for the past seven plus years to do this job, yet we had only been living this medical life for seven weeks. However, we were the ones that saw her every second of every day, we got to know her noises, her cues, her upsets and her reactions. Sadly at that hospital it's more of a fight than it should ever be, two teams working against each other rather than being on the same side. Thankfully we have the other hospital,

I only wish the ambulance would take her there when an emergency arises.

Jovie's named consultant at the main hospital - the nice hospital, is Nick. He is a neurologist and he first met Jovie in NICU. I think he sussed Chris and I out pretty early on, he knew we were parents that weren't willing to take a back seat and we needed to be involved in every decision regarding our daughter, and thankfully he seemed very good at allowing that to happen. Nick is different to other doctors, to start with he has always just been Nick, not Doctor so and so and he didn't do the whole I'm big your small, I'm right your wrong thing. It was obvious he was a father himself as he actually cared, like genuinely cared. It immediately felt like we were part of the same team and he just understood us and we understood him. We all had the same path we wanted to take and that was to give Jovie the best chance at life she deserved, without pushing her too far. We have always said Jovie will be the one to tell her own story and Nick quickly learnt not to presume or expect anything, Jovie has done things her own way right from the start and continues to prove him wrong on many occasions. This is the great thing about Nick, he never pretends to have all of the answers and if he gets it wrong or something doesn't work out as expected, he is honest about it. That is all we can ever ask for, after all Jovie is certainly unique, there are no textbooks about Jovie and she is a learning curve for everyone. Nick also never dictates, his opening lines are always "How do you think Jovie is? What do you want to do about this?" and he actually listens and appreciates that as her parents we know her the best. I remember not long ago he called me from home to see how Jovie was getting on, he was on another period of annual leave and told me how he was potty training his own little boy that week. It's these moments of humanization, of real life, that have helped build the great doctor / patient parent relationship we have and that have allowed us to trust him with our daughter's life.

Getting Jovie through day to day life really is a team effort and another key person in Jovie's team is Shelly. I literally have no idea where we would be without her. Shelly is Jovie's community nurse who visits us several times a week at home. She's the one that really does see it all, the chaos, the tears, the tiredness, the leaky boobs, the seizures, the messy house! For the first few weeks I tried to keep up the pretence that I had it all together, but this didn't last long and she soon saw the real us. She never judges, she's never short of a hug for me or Jovie and in what has become quite a lonely medical world, she has become my shoulder to cry on. But on top of all that, she is the most incredible nurse, who has a brain for remembering numbers and SATS like I have never seen before and she knows Jovie inside out. Whilst we have become Jovie's advocate, she has become ours. With so many medical professionals in Jovie's team, from GPs, chemists, neurologists, dieticians, physiotherapists, radiographers, the list in endless - she is the one that keeps everyone doing what they should be doing and making sure it all runs smoothly. Everyone needs a Shelly in their life!

THE HIGHS AND THE LOWS

5th June 2021
All week Jovie has been so unsettled and screamed for most of the night with no way to comfort her… but this morning we wake happy and rested as our amazing little lady slept all night in her own crib! (We still fed her 3 hourly). Not only that, at her 10pm feed she took a massive 60ml from a bottle (normally 15ml on a good day).
Lets hope we are turning a corner, but for now we are just happy to take what we can.

9th June 2021
By a true miracle our little girl who was deemed "incompatible with life" is 10 weeks old today and weighing 4.14kg, we are so proud she is ours and of how she is showing the world babies like her are worth fighting for. We love you Jovie xxx

11th June 2021
MILESTONE ALERT! Super proud Mummy and Daddy this morning. Jovie took her whole 4am 80ml feed solely from a bottle, she managed a nice big burp in the middle and even kept most of it down. Normally she will do anywhere between 0 – 30ml and that's only when she is really awake and wanting it. Well done Jovie!

On 18th June Jovie had a routine outpatient appointment at the main hospital with the endocrinologist, the doctor that is responsible for keep all of Jovie's levels in check. Things like growth, weight, sodium and temperature, which in a neurotypical body are all controlled by the brain. Due to Jovie's condition of Semi-Lobar Holoprosencephaly she is missing the control centre of her brain, this is what makes her so medically complex. Like a lot of children with this condition, Jovie has Diabetes Insipidus – the inability to control her sodium levels. Until Jovie, I had no idea this was even a thing, no clue that sodium levels played such a massive part on the body and absolutely no understanding of how hard they are to medically control.

On the lead up to this appointment Jovie's seizures had been becoming increasingly worse, and at our visit to the hospital it was decided that she should stay in for some monitoring. England were playing in the World Cup this day and Chris had bought Jovie her own football kit to wear with "MANNING" on the back, he had planned to snuggle up with her on the sofa to watch the game. We were starting to get used to things not going to plan! Whilst on the ward, Jovie had a cluster of bad seizures which didn't seem to want to stop on their own, so she was given a rescue medication called Midazolam. As a precaution they stopped her feeds and put her on an intravenous drip, the first one she had ever had. It took eight attempts to get the cannula in to her little veins.

The night didn't get any better and Jovie was in a constant state of seizure throughout. Despite the seizures not causing her any respiratory problems, she was given another dose of Midazolam to try and allow her to get some sleep. As a mother, it is the hardest thing in the world watching your child go through all of this and not be able to take it away for them. The best I could do was curl up beside her in her cot, stroke her hair and hold her hand. It was now the weekend and Nick wasn't on shift, so we were having to entrust our precious daughter's life to strangers.

19th June 2021

If there was a time for everyone's positive thoughts for Jovie, it is now. It has got to the point where the next step will be taking her to theatre to intubate her and move her to GOSH or Addenbrookes, it was almost already done but she stabilized a little so we have made the decision to wait. The sodium levels are dangerously high, higher than they have seen in a long time in anyone. This is the scariest moment in her journey so far, if they intubate there is no saying she will ever come back round because of her brain condition. So we just need to hope and pray that as her meds wear off her seizures do not return as bad as they were and her sodium slowly comes down and that she is able to maintain good airways on her own. Luckily we have both been allowed to stay with her today, I could never do this on my own, this is beyond terrifying.

20th June 2021

When my eyes won't stay open anymore, they close and I see a circle of angel babies that we have learned of and loved throughout our journey, they are holding hands circling above our baby girl, looking after her and telling her she's not fighting on her own. Baby Athy, baby Noah, baby Isabelle, Princess Aurora, baby Emilie and all the others who have come into our journey along the way, with every thought of Jovie you are all there in my heart too. She's going to keep fighting for all of you, please keep her safe.

21ˢᵗ June 2021
Sitting in the hospital looking at you,
Feeling everything you are going through,
Asking myself did we make the right choice,
Of choosing life, of giving you a voice?
The pregnancy was hard but this is even tougher,
I don't want you to hurt, I don't want you to suffer.
When do we know when enough is enough?
When do we know when you're done being tough?
I will go through anything as having you is enough for me,
I just want you to be happy, comfortable and pain free.
I think about our playtimes and our visits to the wood,
I remember the hard times are outweighed by the good.
Our time at home was amazing and complete,
I pray this is just a wobble and not our defeat.
You took that first breath and you chose you wanted to live,
So whilst you're still breathing you can have all I've got to give.
I am your Mumma and will stay by your side,
And you are my Bubba, my ultimate pride.
With Daddy we are going to fight this together,
And live your best life for the rest of your forever.

We got through the weekend, emotionally and physically exhausted. I think overall we thought Jovie was coming out the other side, maybe we were just kidding ourselves or maybe we just didn't know the full extent of the situation as no one was being honest with us, or maybe they didn't even know what was happening themselves. It was now Monday morning and Chris even left to go back to work, he would have never had done that if we knew what was about to come.

Nick arrived later in the day, the first time he had seen Jovie since he left her on the Friday. Even though the other doctors had been in touch with him throughout the weekend, like us I think he thought she was improving and I don't think he realized what he was walking into. As he looked at Jovie he didn't need any words as his face just said it all, *what the fuck has happened to her?* Though always too professional and polite to use those words. Jovie's body had ballooned to look like the Michelin man, she had blisters over her feet where so much fluid had been pumped into her; but with none coming out it had nowhere else to go. I guess we had noticed Jovie getting more swollen over the weekend but as we were with her constantly maybe the progression wasn't quite so obvious. This would also explain the scan she had over the weekend showing she had Hydrocephalus – fluid on the brain, something she had never had before. Nick turned to me and asked where Chris was. I explained he had gone back to work, his reply, "He needs to come back, now." I now knew something was seriously wrong.

Waiting for Chris to get back seemed to take forever. They did more tests and it gave Nick time to fully review what had been happening. At about 4pm, with Chris now back at the hospital, we were sat down and told by Nick how very poorly our baby girl was. Her sodium levels were out of control, reaching highs of 186, higher than they had ever seen in anyone before. She just wasn't making sense to them. It turned out that an everyday hospital procedure of placing an IV drip, was killing our baby girl. Whilst they weren't to know that she wouldn't react like a *normal* baby, they also didn't stop it when they realized she was retaining fluid, stopping urinating and having rapidly rising sodium levels. Due to her Diabetes Insipidus Jovie's body just couldn't manage the solution of IV fluid. In the gentlest way he could, Nick told us it was likely we only had hours left with our baby girl and he gave us three options. Firstly, we could choose to do nothing, just make her comfortable and sit and hold Jovie until she passed away in our arms. Secondly, we could let them intubate her, get her transferred to a bigger hospital about two hours away, with a paediatric intensive care unit and put her on full life support. Or lastly, they could put a catheter in to help drain some of the retained fluid, give her an albumin infusion and just pray that Jovie was not ready to give up yet. We were basically being asked to choose life or death for our baby. As said previously, we always promised Jovie and promised each other that we wouldn't push her too far, but when you know the alternative to full life support is her dying then it feels an almost impossible decision to make. We asked Nick if he was hopeful of the third choice working, he was completely honest with us and said it was incredibly slim. We then asked him the chance of her ever coming off life support and again he said it was slim. We had been through a rollercoaster journey with Jovie up to this point, but this really was something else. Even though we lived that moment, writing it now just feels impossible to comprehend. Knowing we were running out of time a decision had to be made quickly. Through tears and pain we knew we had to do what was best for Jovie, and life support wasn't it. If she was to pass away we didn't want it to be with a tube down her throat, hooked up to machines and not knowing her Mummy and Daddy were with her. So with a heart that was shattering into a million pieces as we spoke, we asked them to insert the catheter and give her the albumin. We are not religious, but in that moment we prayed, we prayed so hard to whoever might hear us, we prayed for a miracle but most of all we prayed for peace for our baby girl.

With everything done that they could do, I climbed into Jovie's cot and just held her. Holding her felt like the moment it did when she was first born, suddenly needing to take in every tiny piece of her, every smell, every touch, every hair on her head, before she would be cruelly taken away from us. We took it in turns to hold her, read her stories and sing her songs. We took photos of us with her knowing that they were likely to be our last. We told her how proud of her we were, how grateful we were that she had already given us so much and that we wouldn't have changed her for the world. We told her we loved her and we told her if she was too tired to fight anymore then that was ok and she could go. As I write this my eyes are full of tears as I feel every emotion I felt in that moment, I never knew your heart could physical hurt but it can, and it's the worst most heart wrenching pain you can ever imagine. It was almost like the last bit of pregnancy all over again counting down the last minutes we thought we had with our baby, only this time it was a million times worse because she was now here, she had become the biggest part of our lives and we loved her so deeply. We were not ready to say goodbye. The only consolation was that Jovie slept through it all, she wasn't in any pain and she just looked so peaceful.

The few hours that we were prepped to be her last passed us by, then a few more, and a few more. Jovie was still with us, still fighting and still showing the world she was not ready to give up. Slowly but surely over 36 hours, Jovie was back to bossing life! She was still needing a bit of oxygen and her numbers were still making no sense to the doctors but we definitely got our Jovie back. She even managed to have her England football kit on and watch a bit of football with Daddy. We always knew how strong she was, but coming back from the edge of death after her body had undergone such trauma, was something of a miracle, we had one incredible little girl on our hands. Nick realised it was best not to second-guess Jovie any more as she had her own plans for life.

Jovie survived and so the conversation remained unspoken about the doctors' delay on acting upon what was happening to Jovie over that weekend. However, Nick did say to us, in no uncertain terms, was she ever to have an IV drip again – and that was enough acknowledgement for us. Our hearts were full of such gratitude that Nick saw her when he did and gave us enough honesty to stop it ever happening again, that we didn't have enough space in our hearts for resentment.

24th June 2021

Good morning world! I am back to my usual pampered princess status, in Mummy's arms having cuddles on her bed and getting one of my favourite head massages. I can't wait to go home to see my big brothers and sisters. Love from Jovie xxx

Chris - All I hear is people saying it's coming home it's coming home, I'm not interested in that rubbish because what matters now is
JOVIE IS COMING HOME
SHE'S COMING HOME
SHE'S COMING
JOVIE'S COMING HOME
Can't tell you guys enough how happy and excited I am #jovieisaboss

We were back home and living life in full swing, not taking a single moment for granted. Just two days after coming out of hospital, we took a family trip to the zoo. Surrounded by her brothers and sisters, Jovie was back to living her best life.

30th June 2021

A week ago we thought we were going to lose her but today she is 3 months old and is better than she has ever been. Jovie's seizures are at a minimum, she is more awake and alert than ever and we really feel like we have brought a different baby home from the hospital. I'm sure her seizures will creep back in but for now, we are taking this new Jovie and rolling with it – she is still very nocturnal but you can't win them all. Thankfully she has an amazing Daddy that however tired still manages to see to her throughout the night, I really try but I am utterly useless when I'm tired!

2nd July 2021

This is so worthy of a middle of the night post! This girl just keeps on amazing me, I am so so proud of her right now. She just took a full 100ml feed from a bottle, no problem – cleft? What cleft? This girl is not going to let her disabilities define her, I know that already.

Right when we feel we are getting on top of things and starting to understand what works and doesn't work for Jovie, she decides to throw something else in the mix. Reflux was becoming an increasing problem. Despite the hospital admission and serious lack of sleep, I was still managing to pump to make sure Jovie remained exclusively breastfed. However, it was becoming apparent that maybe she was intolerant to something in my milk. I started cutting various things out of my diet, including dairy (the lack of chocolate almost killed me!)

to see if it made any difference. It was a lot of trial and error and the problem with breastfeeding is, it can take a while to get it out of your system, and it was time we just didn't have. I know a lot of babies have reflux problems, but for a baby with Diabetes Insipidus it brings a whole host of other problems. So on 4th August, we made the heartbreaking decision to give her her first ever formula feed, it absolutely broke my heart for more reasons than one. It was against everything I stood for, breast milk is its own magic medicine and it felt so good knowing I was giving her the best I could. But with her severe reflux we had to at least give the change a try as her little body needed a rest. She was put on a "free-from" everything formula, it literally contained nothing she could be allergic to. I continued to cut things out of my diet and kept up my milk supply, just in case there was a chance we could go back to it. On the plus side though it meant I had even more milk to donate to the milk bank and knowing I was helping all those neonate babies meant the world to me.

Her Story To Tell

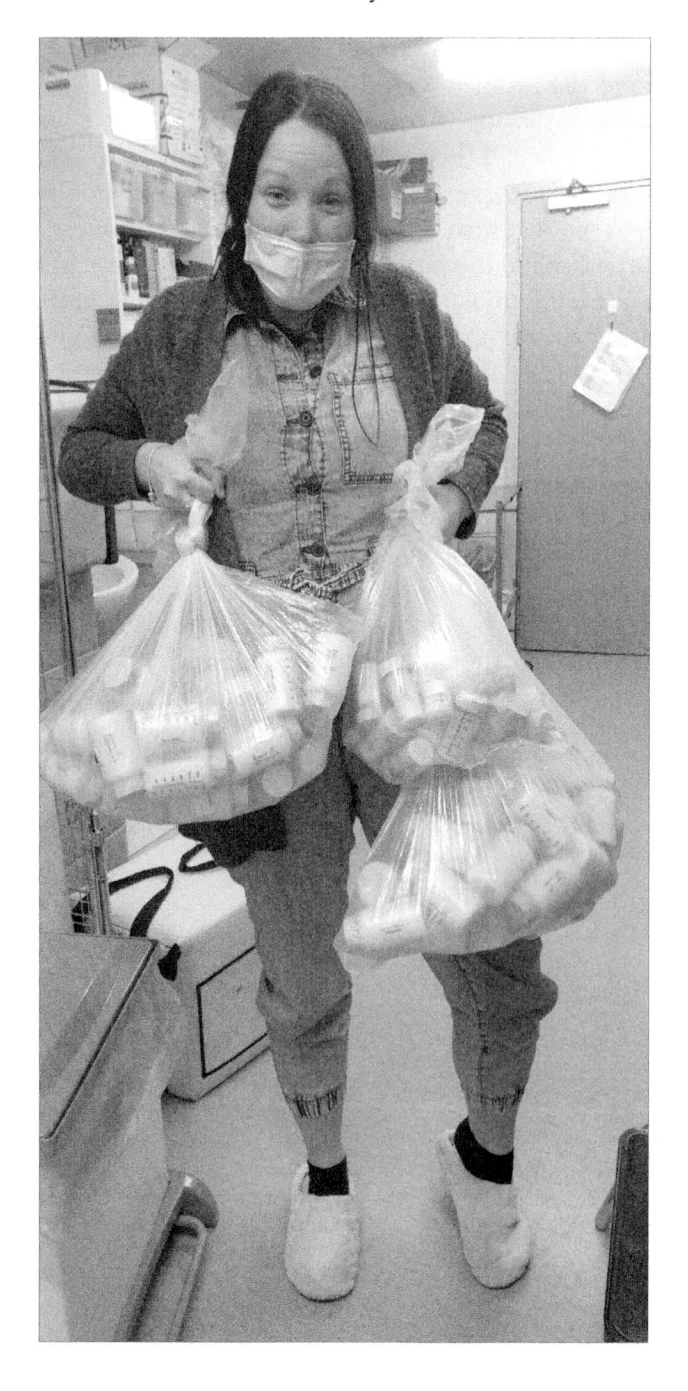

I am fully aware I come across as having a lot of opinions, but they are opinions based on what is right or wrong for *my* baby and *our* family. I never mean any disrespect to anyone else who chooses something different to me, all we can ever do is trust our mummy instinct and go with what we think is best. Breastfeeding in particular has just always been my thing, I love it, I studied it and it was the one thing I could do to benefit my medically complex baby.

The reality of life with a baby that has no control centre in her brain, is a very tired one! Jovie can stay awake for 30 hours no problem, especially at night. Even if she does manage to go to sleep, the intense routine of 3 hourly feeds and regular medicines means we can't go to sleep anyway. With Chris still working as well, it takes everything we have just to make it through a day. This extreme tiredness is something I have never felt before, not even close, I didn't know it was possible to survive on such little sleep. To put it in context, we are lucky if we get three hours of broken sleep in a 24 hour period, and that's been every night and day since she was born. And with her being so complex and her time being limited, there is no way we would ever leave her with anyone else. So we pretty much learnt to just get on with it. Knowing our time with Jovie could be short we also don't just want to survive each day, we want to make her days count. As hard as it is we push ourselves to make sure we are continually making memories as a family and being present for the other children. We have taken Jovie camping, to the circus, the farm and baby groups, to name just a few. Jovie also loves her regular Saturday afternoon watching her Daddy and his team play football – she is definitely their lucky mascot!

Her Story To Tell

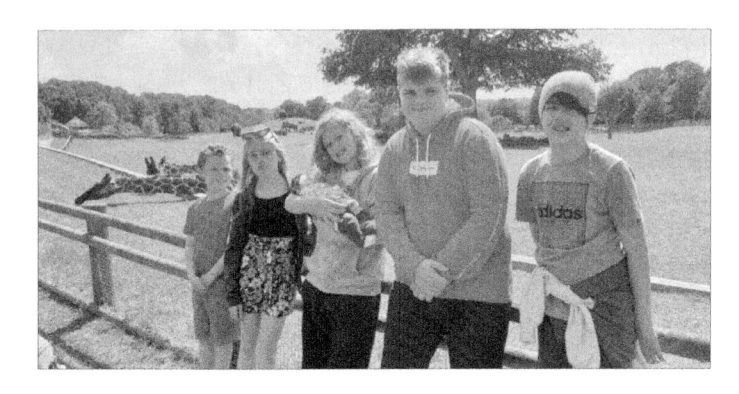

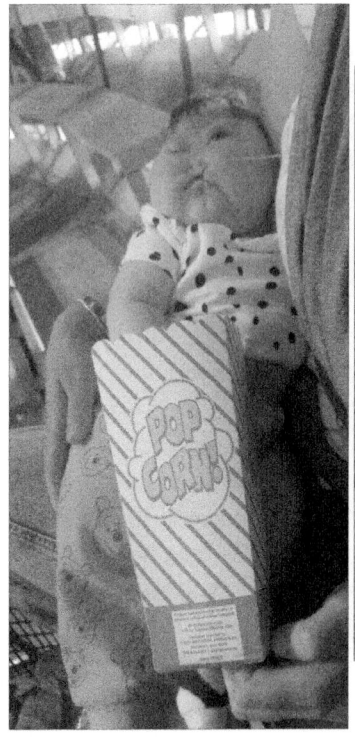

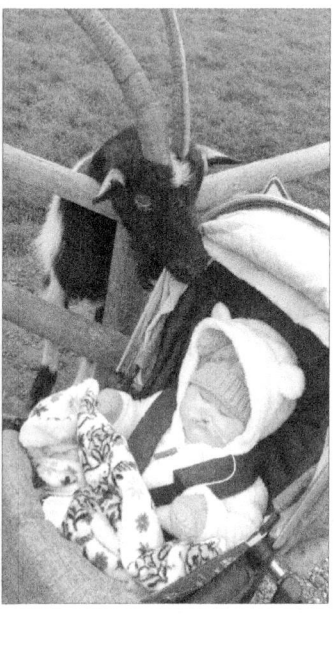

Amongst the fun and memory making, life would throw us a curve ball and on 17th August we ended up taking another ambulance ride back to the hospital, of course to the one we do not like! It was like déjà vu all over again, as they started doing everything that was done the last time which nearly killed her. I tried to tell them, the nurse tried to tell them, but no one would listen to me. I so wanted to be able to trust this hospital and have faith in them but when they will not listen to a mother that has held her dying baby in her arms due to the exact thing they were now doing all over again, how could I? I felt like they were putting poison into her veins, I tried talking nicely then I sobbed as I begged them to listen to me but it was like they couldn't hear me, aside from ripping the cannula out of her arm I was just powerless.

Thankfully after a while I must have made enough noise for them to actually start taking note of what I was saying. It turns out the care plan at this hospital had not been updated since her last admission so they did not know of the previous situation, even though they did have me telling them from the minute we walked through the doors. A different doctor started taking care of Jovie and she was actually really nice, not egotistic like the other, and was happy to consult with Nick from the other hospital, she even offered us a transfer there if we wanted it. But, as she was taking the time to listen to me, really get to understand Jovie and took that bloody thing out of her arm, for once I was happy to stay where we were. I also had Shelly, Jovie's outreach nurse with me all day until Chris was able to come in later, and she is the best advocate for Jovie that we could ever ask for. If only we could have that at every admission to that hospital!

18th August 2021

Not exactly my first choice of where to spend my birthday but it's a day I never thought I would get to share with my beautiful baby girl, so it's still more perfect than I could have ever dreamed of.

We made it home for a birthday take away and a game of monopoly, yey!

We made it back home and in enough time to enjoy our first family holiday. It took a lot of background work to be able to take Jovie a substantial distance from home, Shelly had prepped the hospital local to where we were staying just in case we would need them. It was scary, going away from our safety net and our usual daily visits from the nurse, but it was important to maintain a healthy balance with normal life. Time away as a family to enjoy all the children together was very much needed, and we really did have the best time! Jovie met DJ Ned, won a penguin in prize bingo, felt the sand in her toes and celebrated her big sister's birthday. She also enjoyed her first ever swim, it relaxed her so much she slept through the whole thing! Apart from her first bath in NICU, Jovie has always loved the water. She generally has three or four baths every day, with a couple of them being in the middle of the night. Jovie suffers with muscle dystonia, so the water really helps ease that for her. I then follow her baths with a full body massage, hand and foot rub and body brushing. This is absolutely Jovie's favourite bit of her day (I think it would be mine too if I was ever so lucky!)

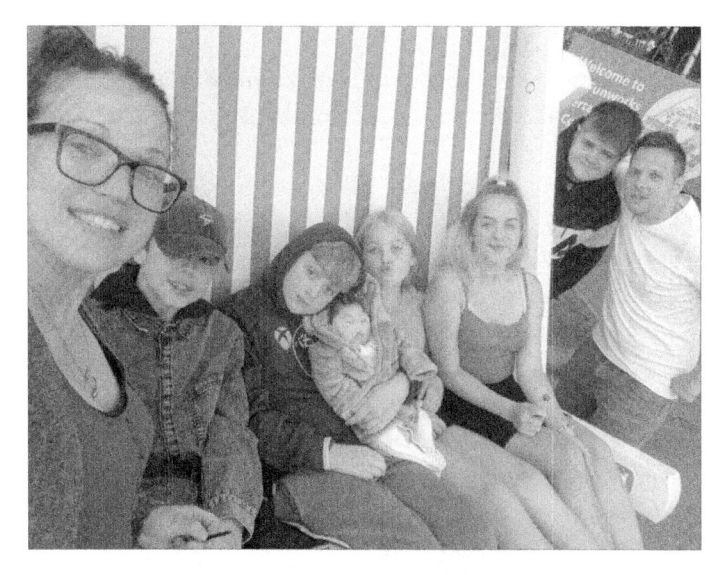

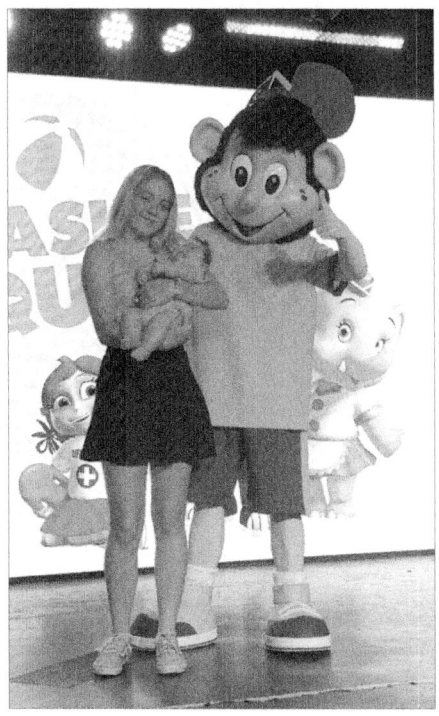

8th September 2021
Eek so excited right now! Jovie has just rolled over for the first time from front to back… This girl can! So proud of you baby girl x

14th September 2021
Tonight I cry the tears of the fears I face every day,
The fears of the time when it is you get taken away.
It all feels too real now it feels like the time is drawing near,
I just don't think I will ever cope without you being here.
I stroke your face, I smell your hair and I hold your little hand,
People try to say it will be ok but they just don't understand.
Going to sleep each night with you right there, wondering if it will be the last,
We've not had long enough together yet, time has gone too fast.
My heart it aches, this pain is real, it cuts so very deep,
I would give anything in this world, if you I could only keep.

Baby girl my heart is breaking, I love you so much.

HALF WAY TO ONE

Every day reached is a milestone with Jovie, we count every week, every month and every first. But there was particular excitement and anticipation leading up to her six month birthday, her half way to one! I am always scared of tempting fate by planning something or buying something for an occasion, but equally I was thrilled to have the chance to throw my little girl a party and I wanted it to be special.

Jovie has the two best little boy friends, Arthur and Hunter, who are about four or five months older than her. I have known both of their mums separately for some time, but they both actually met each other in NICU, so it became natural that we all became a bit of a trio, the babies especially! Arthur and Hunter were both very premature, so between us we have a gang of little miracles on our hands. I love how they don't see any of Jovie's abnormalities and because of her they will grow up embracing everyone's differences and be fully inclusive of others. Arthur and Hunter were at the top of Jovie's guest list for her six month birthday party and cake smash. Not knowing if we would ever make it to Jovie's actual birthday, I wanted to make this one as special as possible. Yellow is Jovie's favourite colour so it took on the theme for the day. I made a massive yellow balloon arch and bought her the cutest yellow tutu with a matching hair bow and a vest that read "Halfway to One". When the boys and their Mummies arrived for her party they came armed with gifts for her and we had party bags for them. We played pass the parcel and the boys had great fun pulling on Jovie's feeding tube and climbing all over her.

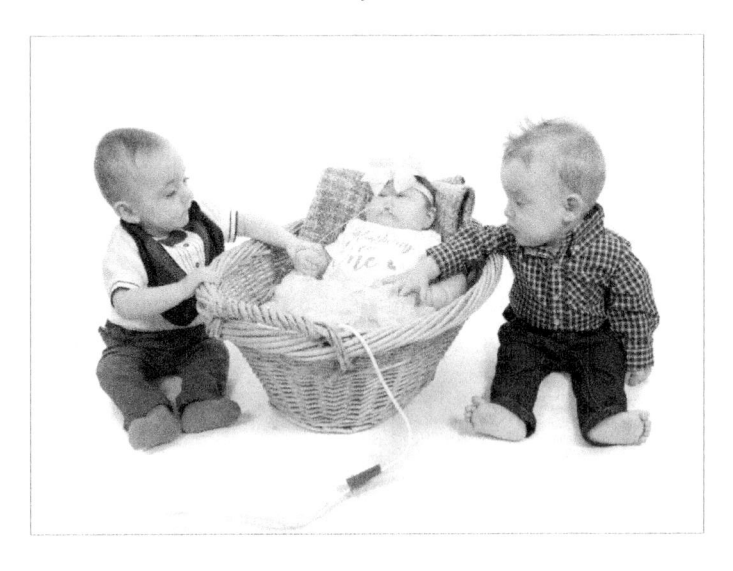

As a professional photographer I decided to include a cake smash photo shoot to add to the fun. And it really was hilarious. I made the cake for the shoot and in my tiredness accidentally used margarine instead of butter for the butter cream. Well it certainly had the desired messy effect for the photos. With them all on the white backdrop in their nappies, Jovie propped in a Bumbo seat between the boys and a big yellow cake in front of them all, the smashing commenced. The boys had great fun covering Jovie in butter cream whilst munching their way through the cake and I managed to get some awesome photos. The trouble came when it was time to tidy up. The margarine that I had accidentally used on the cake made all the babies so slippery, which made carrying them to the bath a bit of a mission. On top of that I didn't even think about the intolerances Jovie has, and the margarine made her all red and rashy, giving me a massive dose on mum guilt. It was certainly one to remember anyway!

Her Story To Tell

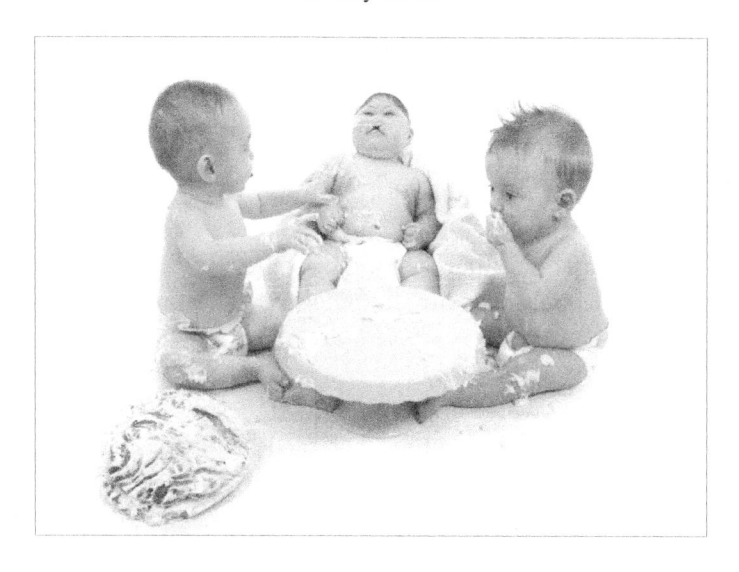

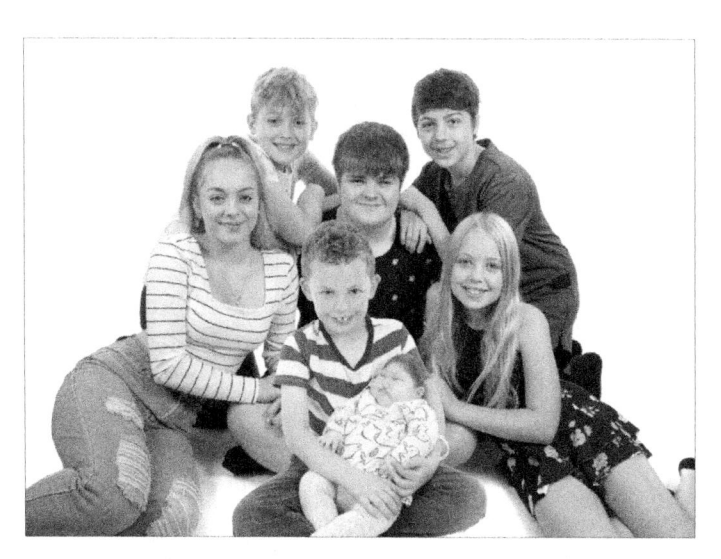

With a day of rest in between for Jovie to recover from the cake ordeal, we then had our family celebration. With all of her brothers and sisters around her (apart from one who we sadly miss), two sets of grandparents, Chris and I, lots of food and yet another cake (professionally made this time – no sloppy margarine in sight) we had another memorable party. Jovie really was and still is smashing life, knowing nothing but love and happiness.

Though we saw an improvement, Jovie was still having some sickness surrounding her feeds so it was decided that we would switch her to a continuous feeding pump rather than her bolus feeds every few hours. This made a massive difference as it meant she could receive it slower. Unfortunately the formula did make her more constipated than when she was on breast milk, so we also had to introduce a small amount of prune juice daily to keep her bowels regular. At least with being tube fed she doesn't have to taste it! It was sad giving up the bolus feeds as it had become part of our routine and it now meant Jovie was constantly stuck to a feeding pump. But it was a change we were willing to embrace if it meant Jovie being more comfortable.

On 5th October, we had an appointment for Jovie's first eye test. Jovie has one eye that likes to open more than the other and she doesn't tend to follow with her eyes, but we never really had any major concerns over her sight. During the appointment I was quite flustered as Jovie had just been sick all over me, so I was trying to sort that out whilst listening to what they were telling me. I think the Opthalmologist was quite surprised how well I took it when he told me Jovie was had significant cerebral visual impairment, and could only see changes in light. It isn't the actual eyes that are damaged; it is the channel in the brain that converts what Jovie sees into images. This means a pair of glasses will never help her. The truth is I was in shock and not really taking it all in. It's only when I got out to the car and called Chris, did the severity of what he told me really hit. It certainly wasn't something that I had expected to hear at all and the sudden realization that she may never have seen or get to see what her Mummy and Daddy look like became really upsetting. However, after the news sunk in, we started to question between ourselves how accurate of a description this was of her sight. We have many videos and notice daily, Jovie seeming to look at us like she can see us. I guess this is something we may understand more as she gets older, but in the mean time we continue to work hard on building her other senses with lots of stimulation therapy. We have lots of sensory equipment and different flashing lights to help with this, and after her vision diagnosis I found a local group called Topcats. It is a group for children and adults with additional needs, where there is an awesome sensory room. This remains one of our favourite places to go together.

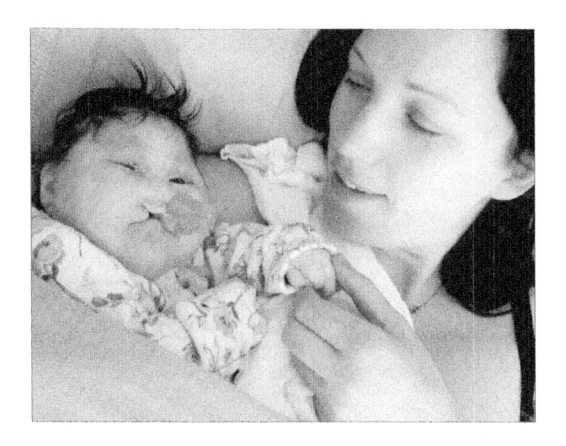

Her Story To Tell

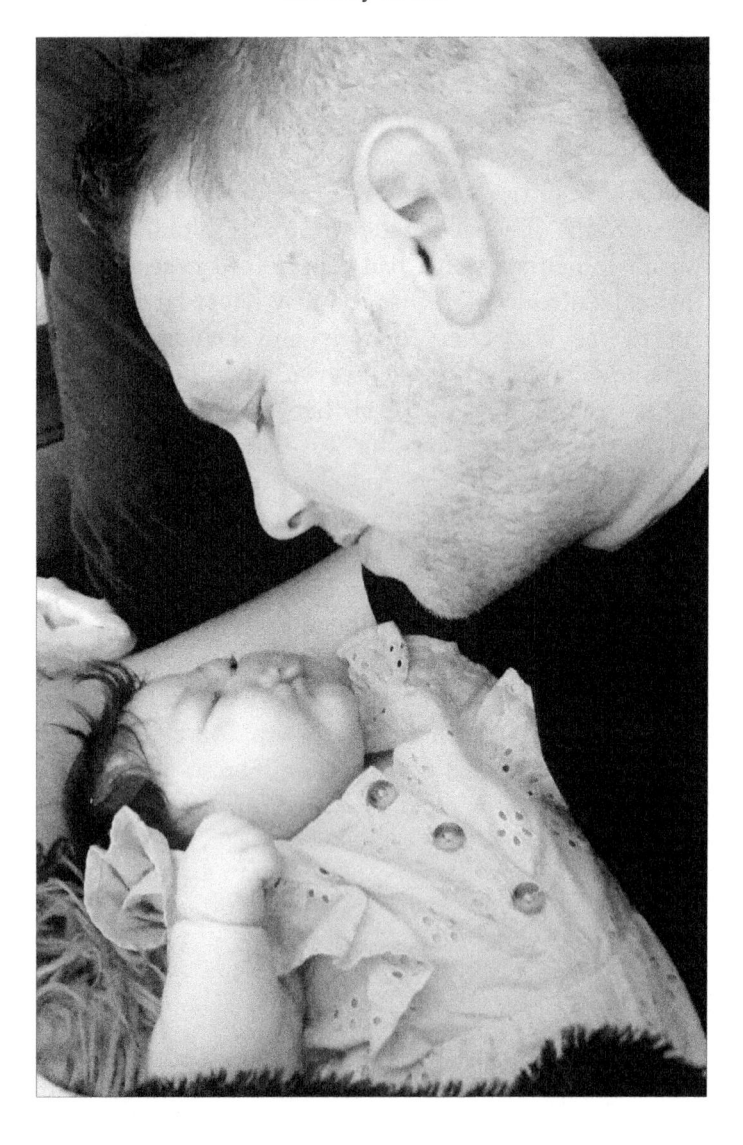

I started to recognize that the daily exhaustion, frequent traumas and the fear of losing Jovie, were really starting to give my mental health a battering. Whilst I try to balance the difficult times with gratitude and positivity, it isn't always as easy as that. In the background of Jovie's care are EACH – East Anglia's Children's Hospice, and they support families in so many ways. I decided to begin counselling with one of their practitioners, just to talk through the things I had already experienced in Jovie's short life so far. With her life being such a full speed rollercoaster, we barely have time to process one thing before something else happens, and it was almost becoming *normal* dealing with these daily traumas and the emotional weight that comes with them. We almost forget that it isn't *normal* to have your baby stop breathing on you, to give CPR, to hold your baby as you wait for her to pass away or to administer rescue medication to stop a bad seizure. Most people don't have to deal with this in a lifetime, let alone in six short months. It felt good to talk about it and have my feelings acknowledged. I continue counselling now as part of my fortnightly routine, sometimes a good cry is all I need to recharge my emotional capacity.

<u>18th October 2021</u>
This girl is smashing life recently and was nice and awake this morning so I thought I would take the opportunity to try her on her first solids… mashed banana! Her little tongue loved it!

A question that is often asked to us is whether we will have Jovie's cleft lip and palate fixed. It had been spoken about a few times with the cleft nurse but it wasn't on the top of our agenda as it would mean a big surgery for Jovie. But on 20th October we had an

appointment at Great Ormond Street hospital, about four hours from home, to discuss it further. We met with a cranial face is
surgeon and a cleft surgeon who spoke in depth about Jovie's cleft. After a not very flattering photo shoot, of Jovie's lip and palate it was decided that surgery wasn't really a viable option. They explained that despite it not looking or being formed in a typical way, it was still working for Jovie. It caused her no problems with her breathing and she was still managing to find joy in taking the occasional bottle and some solid food. They felt that surgery would close up the gaps she was using to breath and actually have a detrimental effect on her. Therefore, the only reason for surgery would be cosmetic and this is something we have never ever wanted. We don't look at Jovie and see anything but beauty, so we would never put her through major surgery where her brain may not even withstand the anaesthetic let alone anything else. A huge flood of relief came over me that the decision had been taken out of our hands, it was certainly not one I wanted to have to make.

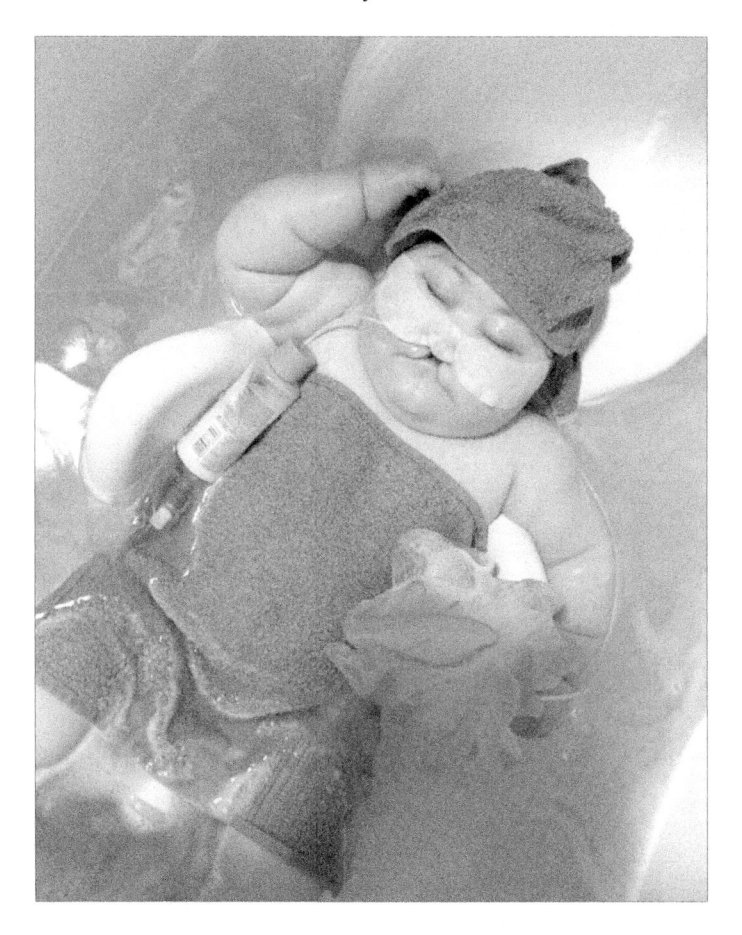

Her Story To Tell

Her Story To Tell

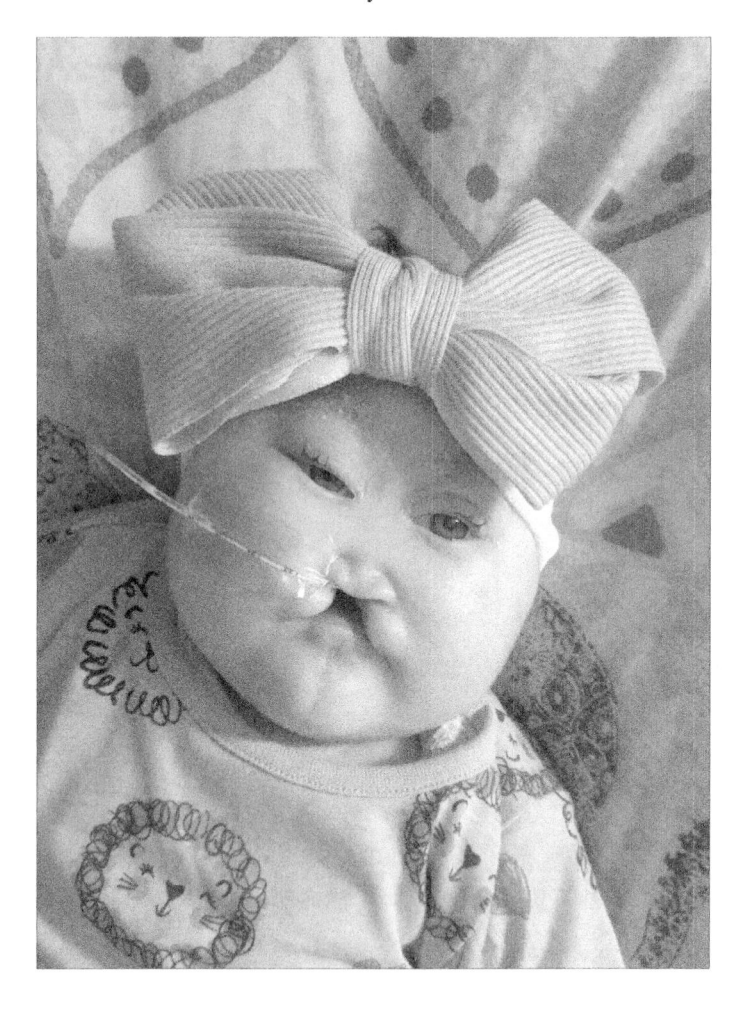

JOVIE'S JOURNEY CHARITY

When we were pregnant with Jovie and found out about her fetal abnormalities, it was never a question for either of us whether we were going to keep her. She was our baby that we had planned and conceived through love, of course we were going to keep her. It soon became apparent to us that we were in the minority and keeping a baby like Jovie seemed pretty much unheard of. We were offered a termination on numerous occasions but our answer never changed.

On our journey through pregnancy and Jovie's life, we have since learnt how much pressure to have a termination other parents in a similar situation have come under from their medical professionals. It has been scary to learn how many parents are guided into an abortion based on the views of their doctor and that doctor's text book knowledge of whatever condition their baby might have. So many parents have told us they didn't realize they had a choice and thought when they heard the term "incompatible with life" it meant just that. But the truth is "incompatible with life" is a term that is thrown around loosely by so many medical professionals because that is what the text book tells them about the said condition. When the reality of the situation is that these text books, this doctor's knowledge, is based on what science makes them *think* this babies life will look like. More importantly, if a fetus is never given a chance at life or chance to develop and grow, then how can the statistics they give ever be correct? The truth is, they can't. We were told Jovie was unlikely to make it through birth and if she did was unlikely to survive the pregnancy, so why when we started doing our research and speaking to other parents given the same diagnosis, was I finding surviving adults with this condition? And they weren't just surviving, they were thriving. This was the case with so many conditions deemed "incompatible with life". So, why when parents are offered a termination are they not given the full story, the whole package of balanced facts, in order for them to make their own informed decision? Where is the conversation that goes "Your baby has abnormality A, B and C which on paper means they are incompatible with life, it may mean that they pass in pregnancy or at birth, but the reality is we have seen adults thriving with this condition." Or how about, "Your baby has a condition which means they are likely to be mentally and physically disabled, but just because this isn't what you were expecting, it doesn't mean their life is going to be any less worthy, fulfilled or rewarding… take a look at this family case study as an example…"

It makes me so mad writing this, that doctors have the power to influence something as massive as killing a life, when most of them probably have no real insight into any of these conditions at all. Again I am at fear of sounding extremely opinionated here and it's probably quite obvious that personally I do not agree with termination (other than in the situation of rape) but that is irrelevant to my argument. Everyone should have a basic human right of choice, but that choice should be an informed decision based on <u>all</u> the facts, not based on a one sided negative opinion of a doctor who *thinks* he / she knows it all. If the parent still decides that termination is best for them, then so be it, but at least they would have made an informed decision, leaving less room for future doubts about the choice they made. My heart breaks for parents I have spoken to, who have got in touch with me after following Jovie's story on Facebook. They tell me that they too were given an "incompatible with life" prognosis and they felt so pressured by the doctor into termination that they didn't realize there was any other option. They then see babies like Jovie, defying all the odds, which then leaves them with a million *what if's* about their own baby that didn't get given the chance at life. Thankfully, and I am so grateful for this, we had an amazing team around us during pregnancy and the fact that Chris and I are so strong minded helped massively. We may have received a few shocked faces and had the odd question thrown at us, but mainly we were met with nothing but adoration that we were continuing our pregnancy.

This void and injustice to parents and babies all over the world just didn't sit right with me. I have just lived through the fear of losing my baby in pregnancy, yet I can still say I wouldn't have changed it for the world, and if I lost her in pregnancy I would still be glad we gave her a chance. And now, I live daily still with the fear of losing our daughter, but again, I wouldn't change it for the world. You see, I wish I could bottle this up and give it to the world to experience; that pregnancy, that fear, that uncertainty of life, my babies strength, her resilience, the lessons she teaches, the kindness shown by others, the closeness Chris and I have because of this journey, the daily miracles we witness, the gratitude for the small things, the empathy our children have learnt and the love like absolutely no other, make every difficult bit worth it, a million times over. She may have a disability but it's that very thing that gives her the ability to change the world. I honestly feel if every family had a disabled child, the world would be a better place.

I realised Jovie was given to us for a reason, and part of that reason is to teach the world the beauty of being different and the worthiness of these lives however short. This realization lead to the birth of the Jovie's Journey Charity and on 27th October 2021 it became an official registered charity (charity number 1196295). The charity is still in its infancy but with our passion it has the potential to grow into something special. It was not founded to tell parents what they should do with their unborn child's life, but instead founded to empower parents into making an informed choice which is right for them and giving them the positive side to an "incompatible with life" prognosis. No one should feel there is no choice, no one should be left with a lifetime of what if's and no one should have to fight alone. The charity is there to offer support through prognosis, pregnancy and the rollercoaster ride though life that such a prognosis can bring.

You can find further details about supporting or getting in touch with the charity at the back of this book.

Her Story To Tell

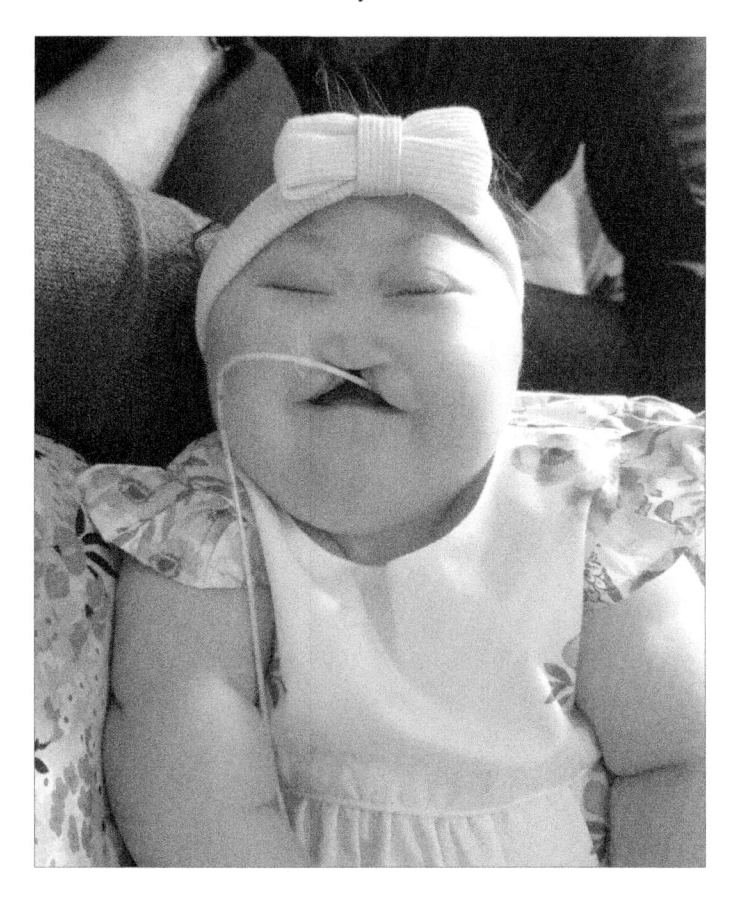

Her Story To Tell

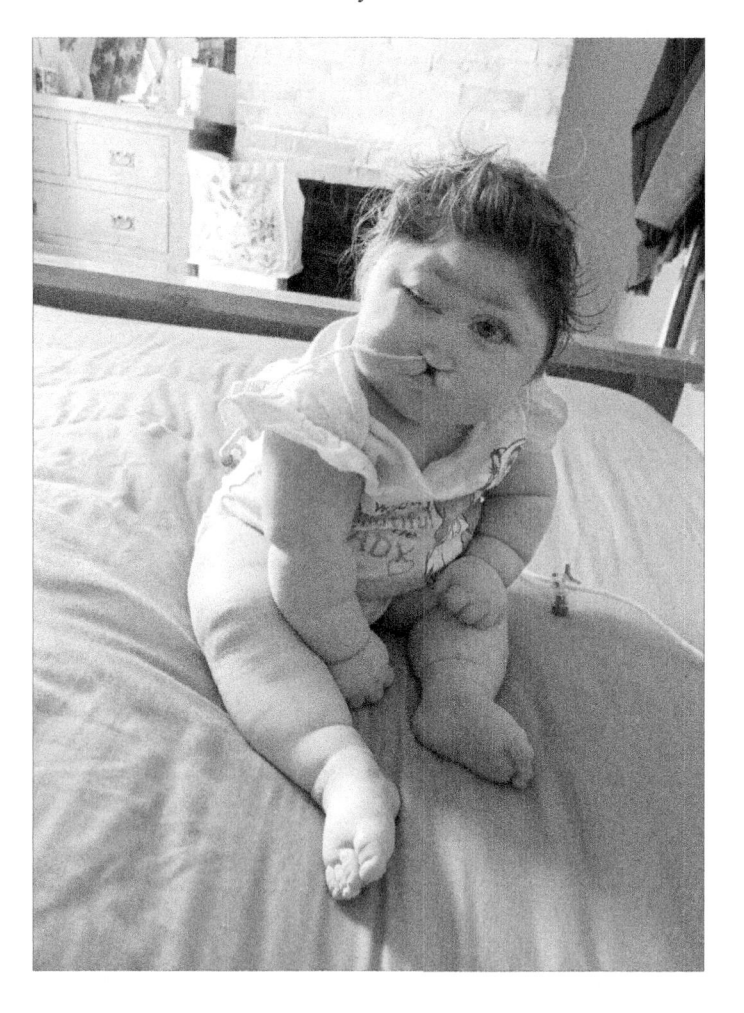

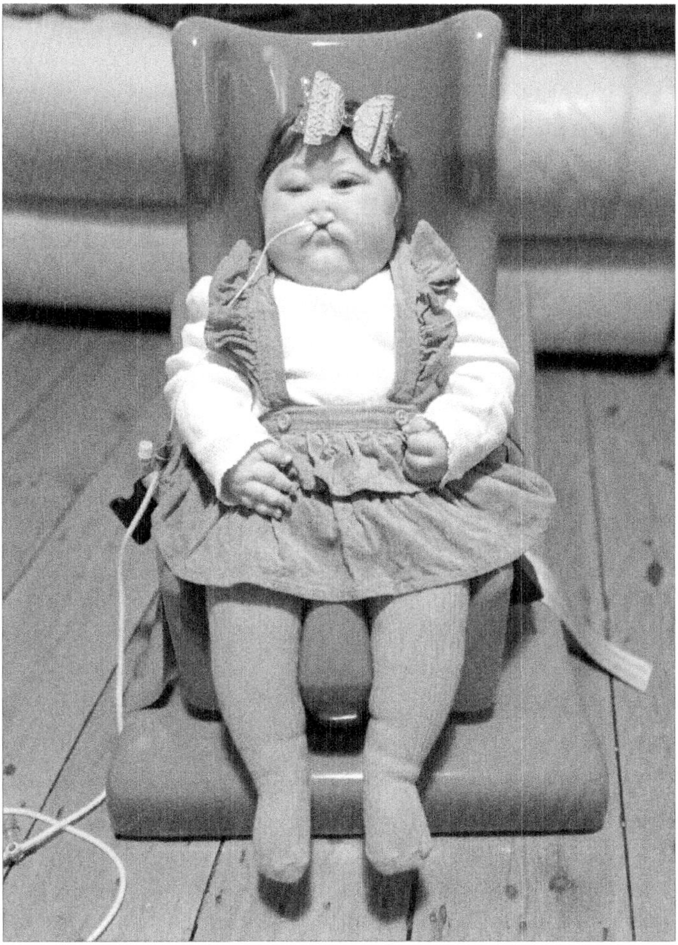

FIRST CHRISTMAS

The months were passing and Jovie continued to fill our hearts with nothing but love and gave us so many firsts, including becoming a pro at sitting up on her own. We had an amazing Halloween where we went pumpkin picking, she took a ride in a wheelbarrow and of course had another photo shoot with her two best boys. With Halloween over, our minds started to wonder to Jovie's first Christmas, a day we never previously dare allow our hearts to dream of. But with Jovie doing so well, amongst the couple of hospital stays that were thrown in (she likes to keep us on our toes), we almost couldn't avoid it any longer.

Christmas has always been a big occasion in our home and one I like to start planning months in advance. I love the build up to Christmas day more than the day itself, with the present buying, pickling onions and Christmas movies all snuggled on the sofa. But this year it wasn't the same. Throughout the whole of Jovie's pregnancy and life, I have tried to only focus on the here and now, taking one day at a time, like never buying clothes that are too big in case she never gets to wear them. Making plans almost feels like tempting fate, and Christmas was no different. On 8th December I pushed myself to get the tree up, it was something Chris and the children were wanting to do, after all, the children were still excited it was Christmas even if I wasn't. It was decorated beautifully with special ornaments I had collected throughout the children's lives, and now we had a "My First Christmas" one joining them just for Jovie. When the tree was almost finished, Chris lifted Jovie to place the star right on the top, it was like the scene from The Lion King when

Rafiki lifted up Simba to show him to the kingdom. It was a special moment we all got to share so I was pleased we did it. But my theory of tempting fate was proven correct all too soon, when on 13th December we were back in hospital.

13th December 2021
You would think we would be excited about Jovie's first Christmas but it's just not something I can accept yet. We have spent the past year fighting the thoughts that our baby is going to die, never did we dare allow ourselves to think we would have a Christmas with her.

We are back in hospital and with her admission a couple of weeks ago as well it's just all too scary to get excited about having her for Christmas. The pressure of keeping Jovie safe, of making the right call, of knowing when she needs more help than we can give at home is just too much sometimes. We constantly live on high alert. Trying to keep everyday life running with work, house, kids and Jovie's needs, and now the magic of Christmas for the other children, it's emotionally and physically exhausting. We constantly run on empty as we barely sleep.

I have never undervalued getting ready for Christmas so much, because right now I don't care that there are no presents around the tree or no food prepped for Christmas day, all I want and would give absolutely anything for is the promise of my baby for Christmas and until I wake up with her Christmas morning I can't accept that she might actually make it. No one should have to live day in day out with the fear that their baby is going to die, but sadly that is our reality.

I'm absolutely full of cold, feel rough, feel impatient and just feel today is one of those days where it's just too much.

Thankfully it was just a few day blip and we were home before we knew it. With Christmas only days away it was about time I put my big girl pants on and got on with some preparations. As much as all I needed for Christmas was Jovie, the children would not have been happy not to have any presents to open Christmas morning. So on 22nd December, we finally got some shopping done and we even squeezed in a visit to see Father Christmas – this was more for my benefit than Jovie's though as she slept through the whole thing! It was an incredible moment, my heart filled with pride as Santa and his elf held Jovie for a photo. You could see they fell in love with her instantly, it really was so magical. Santa gave her a present; an elephant teddy! Elephants have always been Jovie's thing so it just made it even more special, it's as if he was the real Father Christmas!

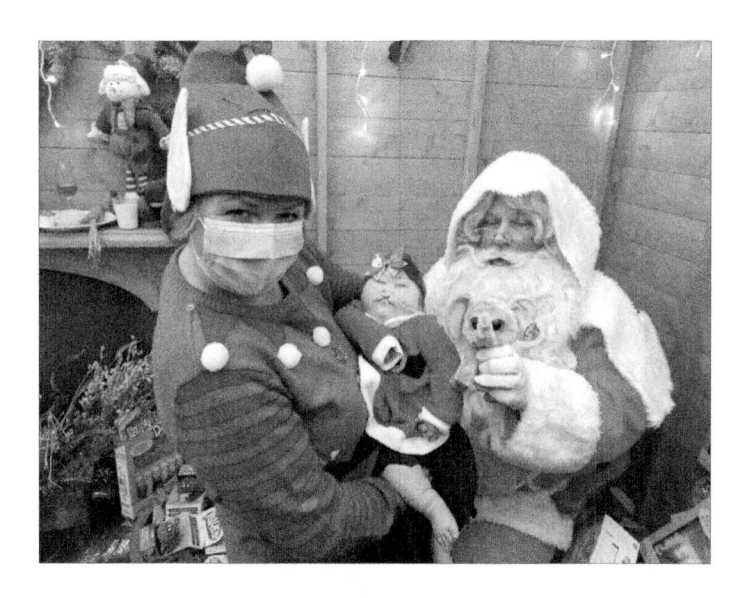

25th December 2021
3.48am, it's actually Christmas Day and our baby girl is laying in my arms and I have the happiest of tears rolling down my face. She really did it, Jovie is here for Christmas, the best present I have ever and will ever have in my entire life. Merry Christmas my beautiful Jovie, thank you for being mine.

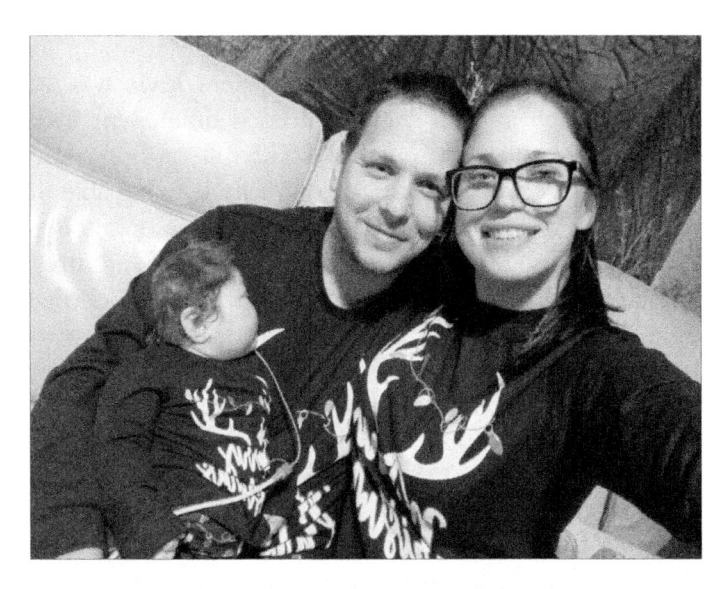

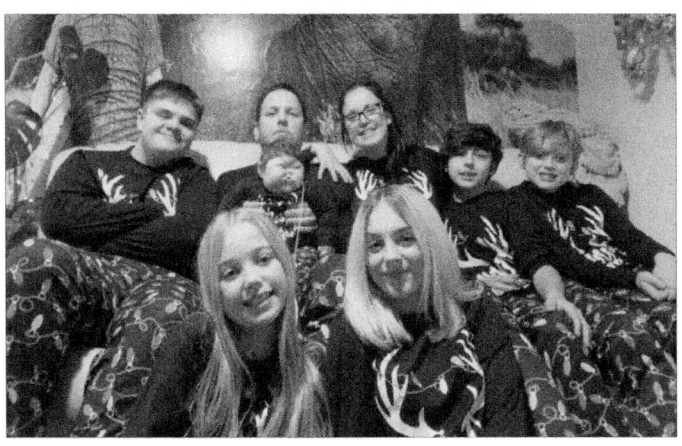

A NEW YEAR

<u>31st December 2021</u>
Our little miracle is nine months old today! 2021 has been full of amazing memories and so many firsts that we never thought we would see… Here's to 2022, hopefully it will bring us a first birthday, lots more memories and hopefully a year full of seconds!!!

After such an amazing Christmas where Jovie was so well in herself and after much needed time spent with the whole family, we entered 2022 full of hope and optimism. We were awaiting news of Jovie being able to start a ketogenic diet trial, something we had been pushing a long time for. Due to her having drug resistant epilepsy we were really hopeful that this may be the answer. We were also pushing for a full review of Jovie's medicines as it was always in the back of our minds that being on such a cocktail of drugs long term, wasn't ideal and could lead to its own problems. We were going into 2022 with a plan and a new found energy.

Our optimism quickly plummeted, when on 2nd January 2022 we were already back in hospital, and this time with a whole new problem. When I was pregnant with Jovie, the question was always, would she have enough of her brain to tell her how to breath and would her facial deformity allow it? We always told ourselves so long as she could breathe on her own then that was our sign that she wanted to fight to be here. Weirdly enough, ever since she was born, breathing was the one thing she never had a problem with. But for some reason, here she was suddenly struggling to maintain her oxygen levels, but for once with perfect sodium levels and seizures not even really being a problem. However, it was winter with lots of bugs going around and Covid-19 was still rife. We were at the local hospital rather than our favourite one so that filled me with anxiety and dread, fearing she would have been written off before we even walked through the door. And to top it off I was on my own again, due to the one parent rule in hospital.

Two doctors came into our side room and asked if they could speak to me in another room. We were already in a private room so why did they want to take me away from my baby? I never ever left her side unless Chris was with her, I didn't trust anyone enough, especially at that hospital. But they were insistent that we needed to talk, so feeling I had no choice I left Jovie with a nurse. I followed the doctors down the corridor in what seemed to be the longest walk of my life, we entered a room, not much different to the one we had already been in, but this one had more chairs in. Clearly whatever they wanted to tell me I needed to be sitting down for. Just like at the time of our scan in pregnancy when we received the devastating prognosis, the doctor pulled his chair close, leant forward on his knees and asked if I understood the severity of the situation. He went on to say there was nothing else they could do and Jovie was unlikely to make it. What was I hearing? I certainly didn't feel this was the case and I had seen Jovie worse than this on many occasions. Why is it with this hospital they are not capable of seeing Jovie for the baby that she is, instead of some text book diagnosis? The ward was full of other babies with RSV (Respiratory Syncytial Virus), it was winter, these things were going round. How could they be sure that Jovie didn't just have a bug like all the other babies? Or why couldn't they see that it might be drug related again? She had just had a new medicine introduced, Gabapentine. A nightmare was evolving in front of my eyes, they were going to just allow my baby to die when all she likely needed was a bit of high flow oxygen, a nebulizer and a reassessment of her dose. I am her mother, I have been there every second of her life, through every hospital admission and I knew what I was talking about! I wasn't desperate and delusional like they probably thought I was, I wasn't trying to keep my baby alive regardless of what it meant for her. Our Respect form said no intervention for goodness sake! I was just wanting a fair chance at care for my baby that likely just had a winter virus! My life is exhausting enough as it is without having to fight for a basic human right. Had they bothered to get to know me and Jovie, they would have understood the mother I am, known that we have never been ones to push her too far and seen for themselves that this was not Jovie's time to go. I fought harder that day than I ever should have had to for a simple nebulizer and high flow oxygen, the same thing that every other baby on that ward had been offered without a fight.

Thankfully a change in shift brought about a new medical team, a familiar nurse and the willingness for them to listen. The familiar nurse, Rebecca, who I knew from outside of hospital as our children went to the same school, walked in with an aura of *let's just get this shit done* about her. She was like my guardian angel that came to save me in my time of despair. She meant business and she wasn't about to take any nonsense from anyone who put obstacles in the way. As I mentioned Jovie needed high flow oxygen which is delivered through a tube with two little prongs that go into each nostril – nostrils that Jovie doesn't have.

Whilst the previous team saw this as a reason for her not to have it, despite me telling them the DIY job we did on the tube at the previous hospital to make it work, Rebecca just saw it as a challenge to overcome and a learning curve for her. Armed with a pair of scissors and some strong tape, Rebecca had knocked her up a special Jovie style oxygen tube in no time! Before I knew it Jovie was receiving her high flow oxygen and nebulisers and my instincts as her mother finally felt acknowledged.

Four days later Jovie was well enough to be discharged!

Rebecca was an example of one of the everyday miracles I have started to discover since having Jovie. I have noticed a lot of people either say to me or comment on Jovie's Facebook page, "I pray she'll be ok" or "God will look after her", I question whether some of these people are religious at all or whether it is just the go to thing people say to offer comfort. Either way, I never take offense to it and I always welcome any prayers that may help us. I sit on the fence with religion, I neither believe nor disbelieve, I think I just pick out the bits that brings me solace. But what I do believe in is miracles, where they come from however is down to our own interpretation. Jovie has made me realise that miracles aren't defined by the enormity of the act or of which high odds they defeat, but instead how they come to you when you need them the most.

On a different hospital stay, but at the same hospital where Rebecca works, I witnessed another miracle. A play assistant who worked on the children's ward, named Andrea, would often pop in and say hello to us, see if there was anything we needed and bring Jovie some toys to play with. I asked her if they had the book

"Can't You Sleep Little Bear", it was a book I loved from childhood and a story I read to Jovie when we nearly lost her at about 12 weeks old. I got it in my head that as she was poorly again I really needed to read it to her. Unfortunately they didn't have the book at the hospital. However, Andrea went above and beyond her job role and ordered us this book with next day delivery, out of her own pocket, and surprised us with it the very next day. This act of kindness meant the world to me and helped me get through a difficult hospital stay.

During another stay at the other hospital, a wonderful lady named Jo, reached out to me on Jovie's Facebook page. She explained she worked at the hospital we were staying in and lived about 20 minutes from our house. She offered to collect some things I needed from home and bring them into the hospital for me. As the hospital was about an hour away from home it had been difficult to get anything dropped off to me. If this wasn't a kind enough gesture on its own, she also included some new fluffy socks, some sweets and a hot chocolate. If any of you have stayed in hospital you will know how good a new pair of fluffy socks feel! This was another miracle on a day I was struggling to get through. During this same stay we were treated to a wonderful student nurse to take care of us, Megan. I say us, it's Jovie she was there to take care of, but she went out of her way to look after me too. She found time to talk to me, ask how I was, let me cry, but more importantly she listened. She was so willing to learn about Jovie to improve the care she could offer her. Megan became my ongoing miracle during every stay from then on.

Jovie seems to have a super power that brings out people's kindness in abundance. I experience these miracles on a daily basis, that they need a book of their own, but to all my miracles whether I have mentioned you or not, thank you. I try to show my appreciation at the time but you will never truly know how your acts of kindness keep me going through the difficult times.

Jovie really is making the world a better place and I am so proud that she is mine.

Miracles really were needed over the next couple of months as they were more intense than ever. My poor Jovie couldn't catch a break from winter viruses and urine infections. They played havoc with her temperature that she struggled to maintain anyway, being usually on the higher side we had a shock when she then got hypothermia. We were in and out of hospital and on top of that her dystonia and seizures were becoming increasingly worse, they usually do go hand in hand with her being poorly.

1st February 2022
Another night and another hospital bed,
Another blood test and another result to dread.
Another time I left the kids without even a goodbye,
Another lot of tears I can't help but to cry.
Another bout of Mum guilt flooding over me,
Another time I'm on my own without my family.
Another time I trusted that Mummy instinct inside,
Another niggling voice and a feeling that won't subside.
Another fear of being here because this might be the one,
That my little girl decides that her time here is done.

By mid February I felt absolutely done in, Chris was exhausted trying to work full time and support us as well as care for the children at home and in all honesty we were beginning to lose the plot! By this point, Nick knew us so well and our relationship was a professional but relaxed one. I will often email him for advice, send seizure videos or just have a moan, nothing is ever too much trouble (as least he never shows it!) This time my middle of the night email was a little different, I was now that desperate mother and probably somewhat delusional too from the sheer exhaustion. I begged him to *please* book us in for a planned admission at his hospital, I couldn't take any more frequent short visits to the local hospital – where even though the care did get better, we weren't getting anywhere in terms of Jovie's plan. I wanted her meds and feed amounts reassessed and I wanted a date for the keto diet trial, my head couldn't rest knowing there were still other options out there. As reliant as ever, Nick emailed back with a planned admittance date and his words "we will give Jovie a full MOT". In our heart we knew Jovie wasn't doing good and we have always known that our time with her would be limited. Leaving the house on 23rd February ready for our planned hospital stay, I wondered whether I would ever get to bring my baby home again.

25th February 2021
I keep trying to write an update and I just don't know what to write. It's so hard to explain the reality of this life to someone, to make them understand that I wouldn't change a single thing about Jovie and all the positivity and kindness I witness every day, but at the same time it being the hardest thing I have ever had to do. Being away from Chris and my babies and surviving on very little sleep is taking its toll today, I've wanted to cry so much. I know it's only been 3 days but they are my safe space, my happy space and my emotional support. It's been tough in here watching Jovie's constant seizures, the plan means we are having to allow her to get worse before she can get better. New problems have

arisen today which will make Jovie even more complicated going forward. Also her sodium and urine output today has not followed the "rules" taking me back in my mind to the time last June when we nearly lost her. This year has been so intense, I think we have spent more time in hospital than we have at home meaning it's been a constant high alert, that it's now affecting my sleep. Even though I am so exhausted my brain doesn't want to switch off which means I struggle to get to sleep, and when I do, I have nightmares that the nurses are hurting my baby or that she is dying. But I had forgotten how much I love this hospital, it feels safe here, it feels like Jovie is as precious to them as she is to me, everyone knows Jovie, even if they haven't met her before they have heard of her, she continues to wow everyone with her strength. The respect they are giving me as Jovie's mum is truly outstanding, listening to me and including me every step of the way. What's been nice this time is the feeling of community here, meeting a couple of other mums with medically complex children who understand this life, who understand why when we say we would never change our children for the world, and who understand this absolute gratitude for being chosen to be the Mum of such a special child. It is not a life many people will ever understand, but one I try to share the best I can.

As always with any hospital admission, the Respect form is always reassessed. The doctor takes time to go through it with us and check our wishes haven't changed and are all detailed correctly. They want to understand the intervention we would be expecting should an emergency occur. It is a very personal document and what is written in them is different for everyone because everyone has their own reasons for what they decide. Doctors can give their professional opinion and guide you on what they think is fair and reasonable on the life in question but ultimately it is the parents' / patient's decision. Our decision has remained the same throughout her life, we will allow oxygen to assist Jovie, but ultimately she needs to still be doing the work herself. Thinking about it now, when I gave her CPR at home I broke those rules, but I knew then she didn't stop breathing because she was at the end of her life, there was something else going on to affect her breathing.

On 28th February, still in hospital, Jovie had an ok day, some seizures but nothing out of the ordinary and we were still on track with the plan. During the evening, I was on my own with Jovie and she started having a seizure. All of a sudden she was sick and started choking on it causing her to aspirate and stop breathing. Thankfully I had the curtains open and another mum saw what was happening, as she grabbed a nurse who immediately pressed the emergency button, I tried the usual suctioning and increasing her oxygen but nothing was working. She went purple in front of my eyes, in a way I had never seen before. In seconds our bay was swarmed with doctors and nurses, it was a sudden hive of activity as the SATS monitor showed zero and beeped like I had only ever heard on movies, she had gone and I was petrified she wasn't come back. Before I knew it Jovie was being resuscitated with a bag and mask. All I could do was stand back and watch hopelessly as my little girl was slipping away from me, I was on my own, she didn't have her Daddy with her, she could not go now, please no.

After the most intense, scariest and loneliest couple of minutes of life, Jovie was back, she was breathing on her own again and she was stable, for now at least. Things were calm for a little while as Jovie slept for a bit but she soon started intensely vomiting again. She had sicked up all of her recent medicines which made the seizures and dystonia more violent than I had ever witnessed before and it was breaking my heart into a million pieces. The usual rescue medication to stop the seizures wasn't working and they had two failed attempts at getting a cannula in which meant they couldn't administer drugs through her veins which would normally have a quicker effect on the body. They wouldn't try more than twice as they just knew it wasn't fair on Jovie. The next option was to give Phenytoin down her feeding tube which takes an hour to work, but even after the hour it had no effect. It was just utterly horrendous watching my baby girl go through so much, and there was no sugar coating this, it was the first time I had really seen her suffer. I knew we were running out of options without a cannula in her and I was so scared she was ready to give up. Some time during all of this I managed to call Chris. Thankfully the hospital allowed him to come in, but being an hour a way from home he wasn't there quickly. I think it was about 2am when he finally arrived, they had just administered the last option, a tablet up her bottom which smelt awful. It stopped her seizing and a sense of calm was once again restored. Even though I told him everything, Chris had no real idea of the extent of what I had just witnessed and of what Jovie had just been through. In fact, I remember my emotions getting the better of me and to put it bluntly I felt completely pissed off that he came in with such a laid back attitude. He literally had no concept about what had just happened. As much as I really needed him there, I am glad he doesn't have to be haunted with those moments for the rest of his life like I will be.

Jovie got a few hours sleep, only to wake very restless.

This time they thought it may be dystonic episodes rather than seizures so they sedated her to allow her body chance to recover. Due to the aspiration Jovie got a horrible chest infection, which put all other plans or hold, first we just needed to get our little girl better.

When I got chance to reflect and process all the events that had just happened I realized the doctor that resuscitated Jovie went against our Respect form by using the bag and mask. I was extremely thankful he did but it was something I needed to discuss further and understand his reasoning. It wasn't Jovie's usual doctor and he had only met her for the first time a couple of days prior. He immediately put me at ease, he was personable just like Nick, he even sounded like Nick and I could tell almost instantly he really cared for his patients. He got to know Jovie well over the couple of days he was looking after her. After I had thanked him profusely for saving my daughter's life, I asked him why he did what he did. I guess I was questioning it as it was such a far cry from the other hospital's actions where they took the Respect form quite literally and didn't even want to give basic support, and I wanted to know why the difference. Simply put, he explained that he knew Jovie well enough to tell that the episode she had wasn't her giving up and it was just because she aspirated, therefore he felt it the right thing to do. This is what happens when doctors actually take time to understand their patients! From then on we changed our Respect form to include non invasive procedures such as BVM (bag valve mask). That was the awful thing about the Respect form when we first had to fill it in and it didn't really get any easier, if you don't know all the options in different scenarios then how as a parent are you really supposed to know what to choose?

Your child's life hangs in the balance of those decisions.

7th March 2022
All being well this should be our last night in hospital, for a while at least anyway. We got a bit more than we bargained for from this stay, Jovie decided to change it up a bit, scare Mummy and Daddy and keep everyone on their toes, but then this is Jovie, she likes to make sure everyone knows she is here.

We knew we would be leaving with oxygen to help Jovie's sleep apnea, however we weren't planning on leaving on continuous oxygen, but after she suffered aspiration pneumonia sadly we haven't been able to wean the oxygen right off. I'm hoping we can wean off in time as she hasn't fully recovered yet. It's bitter sweet that we have made a step to help us manage at home more, but it seems one step in the direction we don't want to be heading also, but it is what it is.

Our routine at home has just got a whole lot more complicated, one with oxygen but two because all her medicines have been switched to tablet form, as she needs to be sugar free in preparation for her keto diet trial at the start of next month when we have a stay at Addenbrookes. Tablets are so much harder than meds!
This stay has seen Jovie weaned off Keppra and Trihexphenadyl which is fab, however we have gained two new meds, one for her hypothyroidism and one which is to try and help her sleep at night, Melatonin. We also have a sedative should her dystonia get too bad.

We have also increased her fluids which I have wanted to do for months and she has handled it like a boss.

So all in all it has been a successful, albeit longer than hoped for stay. We have been taken care of amazingly and everyone here is for Team Jovie. Jovie is not back to her usual self yet and still has some recovering to do, but it's nothing we can't do at home, and home is her happy place with her baths and lots of fresh air, both things which she can't get here.

So fingers crossed for tomorrow as my body can't take any more lack of sleep!

18th March 2022
I'm sorry when you cried last night I put my hands over my ears
I'm sorry it took me that bit longer to come and wipe your tears.
I'm sorry I'm not always as strong as you need me to be
I'm sorry that I sometimes miss the old parts of me.
I'm sorry that I can seem sad and you have to hear me cry
I'm sorry you have to listen to me ask the questions why.
I'm sorry when we sing our songs they don't always sound as fun
I'm sorry when we read some books I only read you one.
I'm sorry I'm too tired sometimes to be the best mum I can be
I'm sorry I spend your time on earth fearing you leaving me.
I'm sorry I can't take away all the difficult things that you go through
But I will never be sorry for getting to be a mummy to you.

THE PROPOSAL

One thing this whole journey has done is bring Chris and I closer together than ever. Whilst I knew Chris was my forever right from the beginning, seeing the devotion he has to Jovie, the sparkle in his eye when he looks at her, and the continuous outpouring of love he gives to all of us, just make me fall more in love with him every single day. Our lifestyle of two blended families, eight children, hospital stays, fear of losing our daughter, lack of sleep and extensive emotional strain is enough to break up any couple, but for us it has done quite the opposite. I will be forever grateful that Chris and I found each other and that we get to share in this crazy life together, a life that we wouldn't change for the world.

In the early days, during our trip to Poland, I secretly hoped Chris was going to propose to me. We had only been together six months but we were already pregnant and we were in such a beautiful city, it would have been perfect. As you already know, it never happened! In the months that followed we spoke about marriage a lot, we always knew we wanted to be together forever, hence why we decided to have a baby together. After Jovie arrived, I got bored of waiting for an official proposal and in true Deborah style (impatient and in control) decided to start planning the wedding anyway.

We always knew where we wanted to get married, a beautiful barn in Norfolk, next to where we often go camping. It was perfect with its countryside location, exposed beams in the ceremony room and with cows in the neighbouring fields it was everything I could dream of. Unfortunately though, with me not working any more due to taking full time care of Jovie and just having the one wage coming in, our dreams were soon shattered when we found out it was well out of our current budget. Disappointed but still eager to find somewhere just as nice, we started attending wedding fayres and viewing alternative venues. We found a lovely country house hotel, covered in green and red ivy, which still gave the rustic vibe we were searching for without compromising too much on our original vision – and it was within budget! We took the plunge and got our date booked in, 19th August 2023.

Still not officially engaged we kept the fact that we had booked the venue to ourselves. With Jovie needing around the clock care and not being able to or wanting to leave her, I knew my proposal wasn't going to be as elaborate as what it could have been in Poland. I didn't mind though, as all that mattered to me was being able to call Chris my Fiancé. Unfortunately Chris took that quite literally when on 19th March 2022, after asking my Dad for my hand in marriage, he proposed over a pile of laundry! For a proposal that was very expected, that was very unexpected! I didn't even realize he was being serious to start with so I didn't take in a word of the lovely speech he had prepared. And with Chris being as stubborn as he is, he wouldn't repeat it either! After getting over the rubbish proposal, I am now just super excited that I am going to be Chris' wife and I can't wait for Jovie to be our flower girl.

On Tuesday 22nd March 2022 our long awaited visit to Addenbrookes Hospital, for Jovie's keto diet trial was finally happening. The highly trained dieticians had formulated her a very special complex milk, to make sure it wouldn't interfere with her sodium levels. I think it was our easiest stay in hospital ever as Jovie tolerated the change really well. We spent a few days there to help me learn the keto process, how to make the milk from scratch and how to test and manage her ketones. But it was balanced out with lots of fun time in their hospital garden, where Jovie loved the swings and going down the slide. The air was so warm and it felt like spring had arrived, I couldn't help but smile as everything just felt so positive and I was excited as to what the trial could mean for Jovie. By Thursday we were home, ready to embrace the change and get ready for Jovie's first birthday, which was now only six days away!

A WHOLE ONE YEAR

She is unlikely to make it to full term.
She is unlikely to make it through birth.
She is unlikely to come out breathing.
She is unlikely to make it home.

They forgot to mention the fun she would have with her brothers and sisters; at the farm, the park, the zoo and the circus, they didn't to tell us about the holidays and the beach trips she would have, they forgot about all of her siblings birthdays and Father's Day that she would be there to celebrate, they never told us how much she was going to love swimming and her warm bubbly baths, or how she was going to go pumpkin picking and put a star on the Christmas tree, they never said she would achieve *normal* milestones like rolling over and sitting up, they never gave hope that she would be here, four days away from her first birthday, having completed almost a whole year of firsts and now celebrating what was my best ever Mother's Day!

27th March 2022
✓ *First Mother's Day*
I feel the luckiest Mummy alive to have all my children together for Mother's Day. Something I never thought would get to happen again, but it did and it's the best present ever.
Jovie would also like to wish a very Happy Mother's Day to her God Mother Shelly, an amazing lady and friend that we just couldn't do without, we are so happy that you are now stuck with us forever!!

I really surprised myself on the few days leading up to Jovie's birthday. I was expecting to feel the usually anxiety, pressure and fear of tempting fate that have come with any of her previous milestones, but instead I just felt so happy and excited that our baby girl was turning one. There really has been a shift in energy since Jovie's "MOT" and the start of the keto trial, things are looking up. I put this positivity into getting everything planned for her birthday, from ordering her a special birthday outfit, buying and wrapping presents, making another balloon arch, getting some big helium balloons including a number 1 and making her birthday cake.

The birthday cake was so important to me. I have always handmade and decorated all of my children's birthday cakes and I didn't want this one to be any different. Whilst it crossed my mind that a professional one would undoubtedly look much better and be much easier considering I was surviving on no sleep, I just knew I still needed to do it myself. Incorporating all of Jovie's favourite things, it was no other than an elephant bathing in a bath tub, and of course with a hair brush! It wasn't perfect but I still loved it.
As the clock went from 11.59pm to midnight to 12.01am, I breathed a sigh of overwhelming relief and felt absolute pride that our baby girl, who was deemed "incompatible with life" had reached her first birthday. I cannot begin to describe the feeling of joy Chris and I shared in that moment.

The day was a whirlwind of emotion and fun, and we made sure it was one to remember. Starting the day wearing her special birthday outfit, a beautiful floral burgundy romper with matching knee high socks and of course nothing less than a crown with a number one on for our little birthday princess. We were invited to take part in a special birthday interview with a charity called "Every Life Counts" who had been supporting us through Jovie's journey since pregnancy. We were on live video call with them so everyone around the world could share in the joy of Jovie's birthday. How far her joy spread was obvious when for days we were receiving hundreds of birthday cards through the post from people all over the world. It was the oddest feeling, getting cards from strangers, but who from the cards they chose and the words they wrote, seemed to know Jovie so well.

We then changed Jovie into another new birthday outfit, a lovely white top which read "I am one" and some black leggings, making her more comfortable ready to go swimming. We hired a warm private pool, and she got a lovely new white and yellow thermal swimming suit to wear. It is important we plan well for things like swimming as she can still struggle to maintain her body temperature. As it was a private pool we didn't have to worry about her oxygen tank and tube getting in anyones way. We were able to leave the tank on the side of the pool, and have a long enough tube that she could still go all around the pool. My Mum and Dad, Jovie's Grandma and Grandad came with us to the pool and seeing Jovie so relaxed in the water just made us all have the best time.

Her Story To Tell

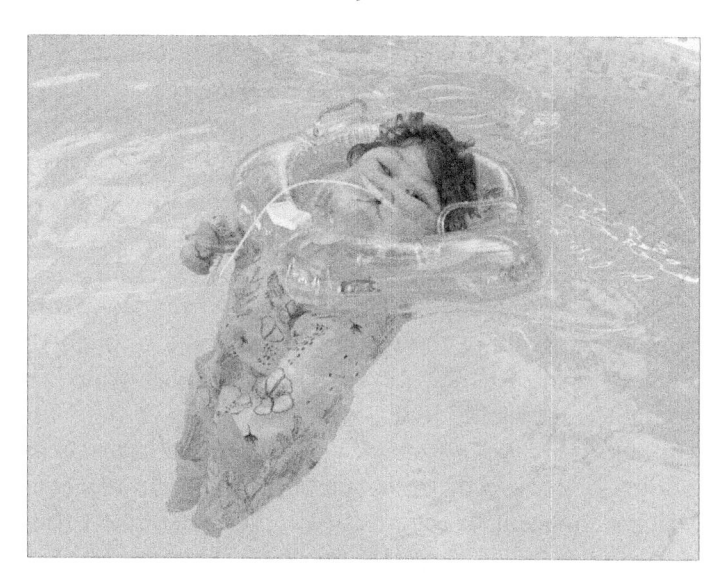

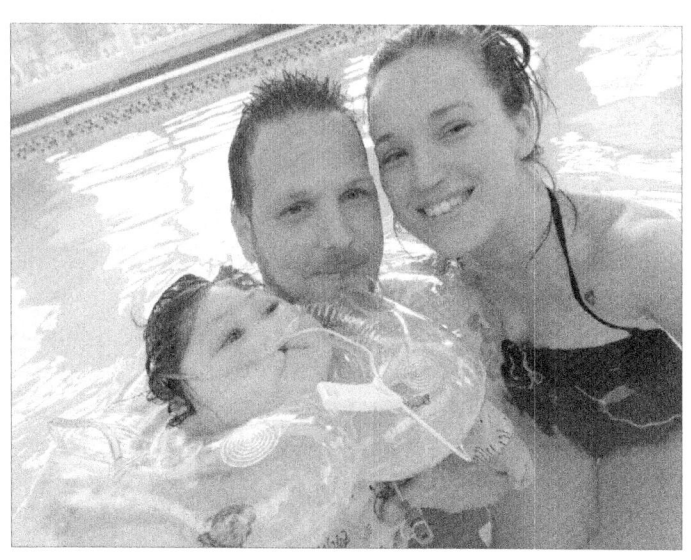

Later on once the children had finished school, we had a small party at the house, where we were also joined by Jovie's Nanny and our good friends Hannah and Grant, who are like an Aunty and Uncle to Jovie. She opened her presents, we sung happy birthday and she blew the candles out on her cake.

Jovie was absolutely spoilt with gifts from so many people, it just shows how many hearts she has touched. One of the presents we bought Jovie was from an incredible company who make inclusive dolls with various disabilities or medical conditions. I sent them photos of Jovie and the result of the doll we received was just amazing. It has lots of long dark hair like Jovie, a midline cleft lip and a feeding tube. I am so grateful we were able to order this for Jovie, but it would be amazing to see more of them on the shelves rather than having to be a special order.

The day was complete, Jovie did it, she is one!!! For the first time ever I finally feel like I can allow myself to have the hope and belief that she is here to stay. Together we are ready embrace a whole year of seconds. Firstly though we had more birthday celebrations to enjoy! A few days later on the weekend that followed her birthday we threw a proper party. We booked out the Topcats venue, the place where Jovie enjoys her play sessions and the sensory room. Being that Jovie has made so many new friends with additional needs, it was the perfect place for them all to have fun and stay safe. Everyone enjoyed playing in the soft play and sensory room, as well as playing pass the parcel. We had yet another cake; a professional one this time which our good friend Ilva had arranged for her, and sang happy birthday. As Jovie's friends all have different abilities we decided rather than party bags, an individually chosen book would be the perfect gift for Jovie to give them as a thank you for coming to her party.

Jovie is one lucky girl to be surrounded by such loving friends and family, and I feel extremely lucky not only to have Jovie, but to know all of the other awe-inspiring, strong, remarkable, miraculous babies and children we learn of, met and continue to meet throughout this incredible journey.

Jovie has taught me that we are surrounded by miracles every single day, sometimes you just need to change your perspective to appreciate them.

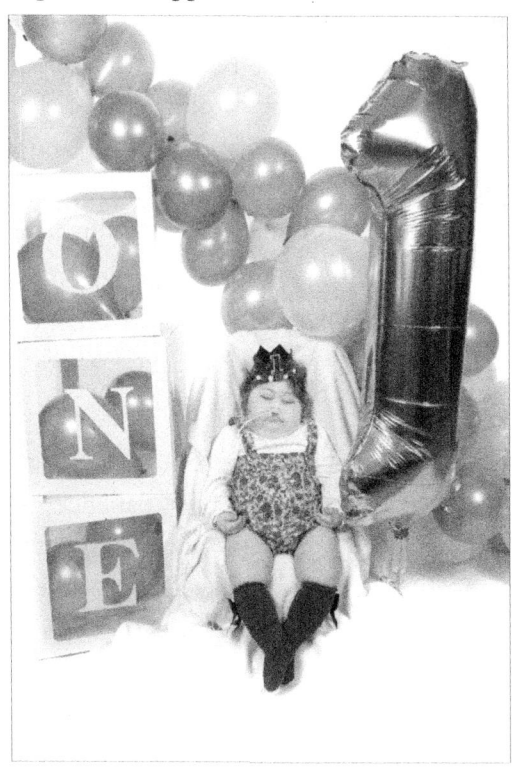

AUTHOR'S NOTE

I always say wouldn't change Jovie for the world. If I got offered the chance to go back to the beginning and be given a healthy baby, I wouldn't take it. I have three healthy children and four healthy step children whom I all love dearly, but it's only when you are faced with the fear of that being taken away do you really appreciate what you have. Jovie is everything she is supposed to be and in her short life so far has taught us more about life than we have ever learnt before. I would choose her every time, again and again.

To Jovie's amazing Daddy, my soul mate and my forever one. Thank you for believing in our daughter and showing the world how proud you are that she is yours. Thank you for being my strength and sharing your positivity when sometimes I struggle to find any. Thank you for loving me at my worst and raising me up to be my best. Thank you for being the best role model to all of our children and helping me to create a home full of love and laughter. I love you forever and always, teamies baby.

To all of our amazing children, thank you for embracing our crazy blended family, for your patience and your understanding. I know it's not always easy when you wake up and find Jovie and I have gone to the hospital again, or when I am too tired or busy to give you the attention you deserve, but you never complain. Just know I love each and every one of you for who you are and for the kindness you show to the world. I am so proud of you all for how you have always dealt with the uncertainty of Jovie's future by cherishing every moment you have with her. Jovie is the luckiest little girl to have you all as her brothers and sisters, and I am the luckiest mummy and step mummy to be able to call you mine.

To our one that is missing and is missed every day. You may not know Jovie but she knows you. She knows she has another big sister because we talk about you all the time. You are included in everything we do in the best way we can. You are loved more than you will ever know, we just hope one day we get to show you and you can make our crazy family finally complete.

To Shelly, thank you for being everything and more, I could not do any of this without you. The only one person in this world other than Chris that I trust Jovie's life with, we are beyond lucky to have you. Thank you for never judging my messy house, my unbrushed hair or my boobs that are so often hanging out of my top when you come round! Thank you for putting up with Chris' terrible sense of humour and our crazy dogs that you are unable to escape whilst just trying to take Jovie's obs. Thank you for turning out to be more than just Jovie's nurse, for agreeing to be her god mum and for being my friend.

To Nick, thank you for putting up with me and not palming us off to another doctor! I'm fully aware I'm hard work, highly opinionated, super emotional and have no consideration for your days off. But I do appreciate you! The respect you give us as Jovie's parents and your willingness to listen does not go unnoticed. Thank you for showing you care and for personable approach but most of all thank you for believing in our daughter and in us.

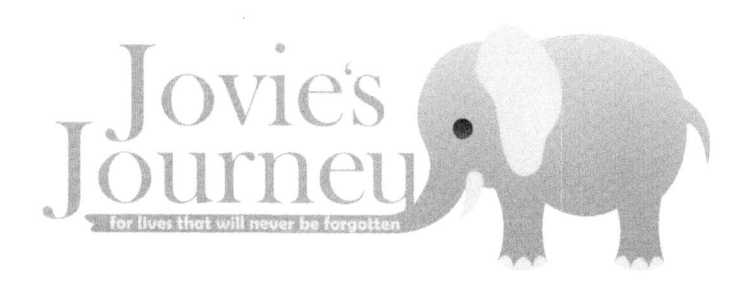

For more information on the charity please visit

www.joviesjourney.org.uk

or drop us a message at info@joviesjourney.org.uk

you can also find us on Facebook by searching

Jovie's Journey Charity

If you would like to donate to the charity then this can be done via Just Giving or Paypal using @joviesjourney